The Veggie Spiral Slicer Cookbook

Healthy and Delicious Twists on Your Favorite Noodle Dishes

Kelsey Kinser

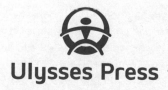

Ulysses Press

Published in the U.S. by
Ulysses Press
P.O. Box 3440
Berkeley, CA 94703
www.ulyssespress.com

ISBN: 978-1-61243-478-0
Library of Congress Control Number 2015937565

Printed in Canada by Marquis Book Printing

10 9 8 7 6 5 4 3 2 1

Acquisitions editor: Kelly Reed
Managing editor: Claire Chun
Editor: Renee Rutledge
Proofreader: Lauren Harrison
Cover and interior design: what!design @ whatweb.com
Layout and production: Lindsay Tamura
Cover photograph: © JudiSwinksPhotography.com
Cover food stylist: Anna Hartman-Kenzler

Distributed by Publishers Group West

Contents

Introduction 1

Chapter One Breakfasts 11

Corned Beef and Cabbage Hash 12

Pear Pancakes. 14

Mexican-Inspired Sweet Potato Savory Waffles. 15

Indian Sweet Noodles with Eggs. 16

Cheese Grits 18

Sweet Potato Sausage Breakfast Burritos 19

Candied Ginger and Carrot Scones 20

Apple Fritters 22

Spanish Omelet. 24

Italian-Style Frittata 26

Maple Peanut Butter Apple Power Breakfast Bowl 27

Black Pepper Grits with Strawberry Jam 28

Zucchini Bread. 30

Chapter Two Soups. 31

Asheh Reshteh 32

Chicken Noodle Soup 34

Pork Chop Ramen 36

Pho Bo 37

Irish Stew. 38

Avgolemono 40

Minestrone 42

Mexican Noodle Soup (Sopa de Fideo) 44

Thai Noodle Soup. 46

Beet Tarator 47

Chapter Three Salads. 48

Great Winter Salad. 49

Anchovy and Escarole Salad. 50

Shuba. 52

Greek Salad 54

Beet Apple Salad 55

Roasted Beet and Goat Cheese Salad. 56

Great Grandma Dorothy's Marinated Salad. 57

Broccoli Salad 58

Carrot Salad 59

Pear Cucumber Salad. 60

Fennel Apple Salad 61

Tuna Salad. 62

Golden Beet with Blood Orange and Miso Salad 63

Potato and Green Bean Salad 64

Chapter Four Sides. 66

Red Pepper Sun-Dried Tomato Dip 67

Latkes. 68

Curly Fries Two Ways. 70

Spring Rolls. 72

Tzatziki 74

Thai Sweet-Pickled Cucumber Salad. .75

Cheesy Spaghetti Fritters 76

Roasted Spiral Slicer "Leavings" 78

Hazelnut Parmesan Carrots 80

Sweet Potato Chips. 81

Fried Onions and Flavored Mayonnaise 82

Pickled Beets. 84

Parsnip Kinpira 85

Zucchini Fritters. 86

Savory Zucchini Bread 87

Chapter Five Casseroles 88

Potato Gratin 89

Mexican Casserole. 90

Lasagna. 92

Pastitsio 94

Root Vegetable Rice and Beans 96

Tuna Noodle Casserole. 98

Chapter Six Mains 99

Garlicky Zucchini with Anchovy and Parmesan 100

Banh Mi Sanwiches. 102

Rice Stuffed Peppers 104

Pesto Pasta. 105

Spaghetti Bolognese. 106

Classic Meatballs 108

Crawfish Pasta. 109

Lobster and Seafood Mélange Pasta. 110

Shrimp Scampi. 112

Chicken Lo Mein. 113

Japchae. 114

Beef Stroganoff. 116

Porcini Pancetta Parsnip Risotto. 117

Paella 118

Pork Katsudon. 120

Mini Greek Turkey Meatballs on Zucchini Noodles. 122

Veggie Patty. 124

Potato Noodles with Andouille and Red Beans 125

Pad See Ew 126

Pad Thai. 128

Alsatian Potato Bowl. 130

Bibimbap 132

Indian-Style Potatoes and Chickpeas 134

Truffle Mac and Cheese 136

Greek Mac and Cheese 137

Sushi. 138

Butternut Squash, Browned Butter, and Sage 140

Quesadillas 142

Chapter Seven Desserts 143

Apple and Oat Crisps 144

Tzimmes 145

Pear Walnut and Chocolate Salad. 146

Chestnut Pear Parfaits 148

Apple Noodle Kugel. 149

Parsnip Cake 150

Raw Fruit Tart. 152

Pear Bread Pudding with Bourbon Whipped Cream. 154

Sticky Rice with Honeyed Mango 156

Conclusion 157

Conversion Charts 158

Acknowledgments 160

About the Author. 161

Introduction

Who doesn't love pasta? No one, that's who. But who needs all those simple carbohydrates and empty calories from pasta? The answer, once again, is no one. What if you could continue to have all of your favorite pasta dishes, from lasagna to lo mein to kugel to everything in between, without all of the refined sugars and simple carbohydrates? And what if you could simultaneously enjoy all of your favorite noodles while upping the amount of fruits and vegetables in your daily diet? Sounds like a win-win scenario, does it not? That's because it is, and with this book, I'm going to walk you through how to do just that while also showing you how to "vegetize" almost any pasta- or rice-based recipe. While this is much easier to accomplish than it sounds, it does involve a small one-time investment in a vegetable spiral slicer.

Vegetable spiral slicer. It's a mouthful for sure and may sound foreign (or at least novel) to you now, but it's really nothing but a big old name for a small new appliance. Affectionately called "zoodlers" or "spiralizers" for short, a surprising number of spiral slicers are on the market today.

Why should you bother getting a new appliance just to make vegetable noodles? Because it's one of the easiest methods to getting more vitamins, fiber, and other nutrients in your diet while simultaneously cutting your intake of simple carbohydrates. If you're trying to avoid gluten or stick to a Paleo diet, I can't think of an easier way to re-create many dishes that would be considered "off the table." I've found that it's also one of the simplest ways to get children excited about making and eating their veggies. Kids love to use the spiral slicer—a big motivation to use it often in my elementary school cooking classes. The average serving (about 2 cups of cooked vegetable noodles) ranges anywhere from 10 to 35 percent of the calories of classic pasta.

It is possible to make different types of veggie noodles with things you may already own, but you won't be able to achieve those long, slender spiral noodles without a veggie spiral slicer. You can, however, make yourself some nice zucchini lasagna or stuffed veggie manicottis. For these styles of noodles you can use a mandolin or a vegetable peeler. If you want to make some sweet potato rice you can use a shredding blade attachment for the food processor or a simple cheese grater. Ultimately, I'm sure you'll find the low cost and high usability of the spiralizer of your choice a worthwhile investment for your heart health, waistline, and taste buds. You can add veggie noodles to soups, salads, sandwiches, use them in place of pastas, and easily surpass the daily recommended serving of vegetables.

Types of Spiralizers

Let's take a brief moment to look over the most popular brands, their pros and cons, and their average cost as of the writing of this book.

The most popular style of spiralizer is the tri-blade, as it offers three different slicing blades to make a fantastic variety of noodles. My personal favorite brand to use is the Paderno Spiralizer 3-Blade, though I have had success with other brands. Currently Paderno offers three- and four-blade options. The average price runs from $25 to $55 dollars depending on where you make your purchase. I personally find the fourth blade to be unnecessary and therefore stick with the cheaper three-blade option. Pros of this model include ease of use, ease of clean up, three different blades for creating different noodles, low cost, ability to spiralize fruits and veggies of many different sizes, and the fact that it's lightweight and easy to store. Cons include occasional loosening of the suction cup feet and seemingly weak plastic teeth for securing tougher root vegetables and squashes (although none I've used have actually broken). The three- (or tri-) blade style of spiralizer is the one we will use most throughout this book. There are other brands offering this style, including the Spiralizer Elite Spiral Slicer, Brieftons Tri-Blade Spiralizer, Benriner Turning Slicer, Kitchen Basics Tri-Blade Plastic Spiral Vegetable Slicer, iPerfect Kitchen Tri-Blade Vegetable Spiralizer, and Inspiralizer from the wonderful spiral slicer–based blog Inspiralized.com.

The second most popular style of spiral slicer is one that resembles a pencil sharpener. The most well-known brands for this style are the Veg-getti, All Times Finest, SpiraLife, Supreme Home Cook, and Gogogu. I'm going to be honest here, while the prices are much lower (starting any-where from $10 for a single blade to $25 for a multi-blade option), I do not find them to be worth the cost. But let's break them down into pros and cons so that you can make your own educated purchases.

Handheld spiralizers are lower in cost and smaller, therefore taking up less kitchen space, but that's about it when it comes to the pros. These spiralizers are more difficult to clean, somewhat awkward to use since you have to hold them, and limited in the type of fruits and vegetables that you can use with them. The size of these slicers are primarily geared toward zucchinis, carrots, and other long and slender veggies. I will not refer to this style of slicer from this point on.

Another option is the hand-crank style that resembles a baby food pro-cessor. The Joyce Chen Spiral Slicer seems to be the most common of this style. I've found it priced anywhere from $20 to $35. It is outfitted with three main pieces: a bottom-level "receiving" area where the noodles are deposited, a middle section to place the vegetable that is about to be sliced, and a blade/crank apparatus on top. The main advantage of this style is that the noodles are kept nice and contained in the bottom portion of the appliance. The cons are many. The machine has more parts to clean, is bulky, requires you to crank somewhat hard, and all of your vegetables must be trimmed to fit into the middle slicing compartment. As an alterna-tive, I would recommend using specialty blades on your food processor if you have one, which leads us to the other methods available using equipment already found in your kitchen.

The vegetable noodles will simply be called noodles. Most of the recipes will be made with a tri-blade spiralizer in mind. The blades will be referred to as blade 1, blade 2, or blade 3. Blade 1 is the single blade that makes large long, wide ribbon noodles, or fettuccine-esque noodles. Blade 2 is the larger of the two multiple-noodle blades, and is great for making your own curly fries or any noodle that would break down easily, like the apples in the apple fritter recipe. Blade 3, the smaller multi-noodle blade, is the one most often used in this book. This blade makes angel hair pastas and is also great for rice recipes, although those get pulsed in a food processor after spiralizing, so if you hate the idea of using two appliances for the job you can get away with using a food processor with the shredding blade attachment.

What Can I Spiralize?

Now that all of that is out of the way and you have a better understanding of the types of spiralizers on the market, let's take a look at the wonderful multitude of fruits and vegetables that lend themselves to this simple and delicious cooking style. The following varieties can be spiralized with a three-blade slicer:

Vegetables

- Beets
- Broccoli (the stem)
- Burdock root
- Butternut squash (the neck)
- Cabbage (works in a slicer, but does not make noodles)
- Carrots
- Cauliflower (the stem)
- Celery roots (celeriac)
- Chayote
- Cucumbers (English or seedless work especially well)
- Daikon
- Jicama
- Kohlrabi

- Onions (works in a slicer, but does not make noodles)
- Parsnips
- Potatoes
- Radishes
- Rutabagas
- Summer squash
- Sweet potatoes/yams
- Taro roots
- Turnips
- Zucchinis (naturally!)

Fruits

- Apples
- Pears
- Plantains

If, at the grocery store or farmer's market, you happen to find yourself trying to figure out if the gorgeous produce in front of you will be compatible with a spiralizer, ask yourself the following questions (keeping in mind you will need a three-blade style for most items):

1. Is the flesh of the fruit/vegetable firm? This is an absolute must. If the inside is too wet or soft, it will turn into mush as you attempt to slice it. Eggplant is the perfect example of a vegetable that looks like it would work perfectly, but is too soft and full of seeds to work.

2. Does the fruit/vegetable have a giant pit? Even though mangoes can be firm, the tough and large pit in the center will prevent them from working in the slicer.

3. Is the part of the fruit/vegetable that you plan on slicing solid? You can spiral slice the stems of broccoli and cauliflower, but not the head, as the florets are not completely solid. You can also slice the long, thick neck of butternut squash, but if you attempt to spiralize the base, it just crumbles.

4. Is the fruit/vegetable at least 2 inches long? Some will say 1½ inches, but realistically, you won't get enough noodles out of this length to make it worth it.

5. Is the fruit/vegetable at least 1 inch in diameter? You need at least 1½ inches to get true noodles out of it, but you can make slaw out of

thinner carrots or parsnips. Anything less than an inch isn't worth it, though, as you'll lose most of that to the core left behind.

Some of these vegetables, primarily cabbage and onion, work great on the spiral slicer, but do not necessarily create noodles. In these instances the slicer works more like a mandolin, also known as a Chinese slicer.

When shopping for "long" vegetables like potatoes, butternut squash, and zucchinis, keep an eye out for the straightest vegetable options possible. If you end up with a curved zucchini or squash, don't fret—just cut the vegetable in halves or thirds to create the straightest segments possible. The thicker the potato or zucchini, the better. With butternut squash being as thick and tough as it is, it helps to go for the thinner ones. Look for the specimen with the least-bulbous base.

When shopping for "round" fruits and vegetables like apples, rutabagas, or beets, look for the plants that are fat and round and as even as possible. You don't want apples that look "slanted" when standing upright on the table. You'll need flat ends on both sides when you load the slicer and don't want to waste anything cutting it off to get it ready.

And lastly, quality is key here, people. With fresh fruits and veggies being the stars of the dish, more often than not, the outcome will depend on the quality of the produce you choose. You want your vegetables to be firm, never soft or mushy. Zucchinis should have a nice deep green color to them and no bruises or soft spots. Fruit should be ripe but also firm. Again, avoid any items with large spots of bruising.

Prepping Your Veggies for the Spiralizer

Now that you've picked the perfect produce, how do you make it ready for the machine?

The first question usually is: to peel or not to peel? Personally, I'm in the no-peel camp. Fruits and vegetables carry so many of their vitamins in the peels, and if you're buying organic, you shouldn't have to worry about wax or pesticides. If you're not buying organic, then I do recommend peeling, especially the root vegetables and fruits. Peeled zucchinis definitely look more like pasta, so this could be good if you are trying to feed picky children or dinner guests, but ultimately, unless the recipe calls for peeled or unpeeled produce, the choice is yours.

Getting the spiral slicer ready will depend on the model you have. Load the blade you want to use. If you have suction cup feet, get those set up as well.

Slice the bottoms and tops off of the fruit/vegetable, line the centers up with the corer on the blade, slide the platform with the crank and teeth toward the fruit/vegetable, and secure the teeth in. You're ready to crank out some noodles! It works best if you apply steady pressure, but if you have any issues where the teeth of the crank are bending, ease up and check to make sure you're properly lined up. This can happen with tougher things like sweet yams and butternut squash.

The recipes in this book do refer to which blade you will need to use. Blade 1 creates the largest slice, blade 2 is in the middle, and blade 3 makes the smallest, spaghetti-like noodle.

A Note on Zucchini and Cucumber Noodles and Water

Zucchinis and cucumbers are full of water that they are just waiting to release, leaving what should be a crispy pizza or thick ragu a soggy mess. In nearly every recipe (unless stated otherwise), I lightly salt my zucchini and cucumber noodles and let them sit in a colander in the sink to drain. Afterward I gently squeeze out the excess moisture and use as stated in the recipe. Alternatively you could cook the noodles separately from the sauce and other components, but that takes extra time. Draining in the colander can be done while you assemble the other ingredients.

Some of the recipes in this book will say spiralized, then riced. This is one of my favorite features of the spiral slicer. Take a bunch of noodles sliced on blade 3 and pulse them in the food processor until it resembles rice—simple as that!

Now you are truly ready to use your noodles and/or rice.

How to Use This Book

Some of the recipes in this book are vaguer than others. They may say "1 medium zucchini" or they may say "2 cups zucchini noodles." Generally, if the recipe does not specify the amount of noodles in cups, then it does not have to be super accurate. Use your best judgment and work to your tastes.

Small zucchinis, summer squashes, cucumbers, potatoes, and similar-sized vegetables will be 3 to 4 inches or less. Medium would be between 4¼ to 7 inches, and large is anything above 7 inches. Feel free to play around with the recipes in this book. You can always substitute summer squash for zucchini or sweet potato for butternut squash, and many of the root vegetables are interchangeable.

If butter is listed in the recipe but does not fit your diet, you can use butter substitutes or olive oil. Some of the recipes call for browned butter, however, and the outcome will not be the same, but they will still be delicious. Feel free to substitute rice flour for the all-purpose flour in the fritter dishes. Above all, stay true to your tastes and dietary needs, and don't be afraid to play with your food.

Recipes

CHAPTER ONE
Breakfasts

Breakfast is my favorite meal of the day. By now we've all heard how important it is to eat breakfast, as it helps you stay full longer and prevents too much snacking or overeating at lunch. It also sets the tone for your day. If you take the time to make a nice, healthy, and peacefully paced breakfast, the rest of your day will seem a lot easier to face—trust me. In this section, I cover everything from a peanut butter and apple "power bowl" to a weekend indulgence of apple fritters.

Corned Beef and Cabbage Hash

Hash is most commonly found in a can these days, which is a crying shame since it's one of America's best breakfast staples. This is a great post–St. Paddy's Day hangover brunch recipe, or just an excellent excuse to get corned beef and cabbage more than once a year.

MAKES 4 SERVINGS

4 tablespoons butter, divided

1 large parsnip, spiralized on blade 2

1 large rutabaga, spiralized on blade 2

4 slices thick-cut bacon, cut into ¼-inch slices

1 large yellow onion, diced

1 pound corned beef, cooked and cut into ½-inch chunks

2 tablespoons chopped fresh sage

1 cup beef broth

1½ cups shaved cabbage, spiralized on blade 1

salt and pepper, to taste

4 fried eggs, to top

1. In a large, oven-safe skillet (preferably cast-iron) melt 2 tablespoons of the butter on medium heat. Add the parsnip and rutabaga noodles and stir to coat with the melted butter. Add ¼ cup of water, bring to a simmer, cover, and cook for 7 to 10 minutes. Drain the partially cooked noodles and set aside.

2. Preheat the oven to 400°F.

3. Return the skillet to the stove, increase the heat to medium-high, and add the sliced bacon. Cook until the bacon begins to release its fat, about 3 minutes. Add the diced onion and stir frequently, cooking for another 5 minutes or so until the onion starts to turn translucent. Add salt and pepper, to taste.

4. Add the corned beef, sage, and reserved root vegetable noodles. Stir occasionally, allowing the ingredients to gather some color. Add one more tablespoon of the butter if the noodles and corned beef begin to stick to the pan. Add the beef broth and place the pan in the

oven for 10 to 15 minutes or until the liquid is absorbed and the hash begins to get crisp. Remove from the oven and top with a plate to keep warm.

5. While the hash is baking, cook the shaved cabbage on the stovetop in a large skillet with the last tablespoon of butter. Cook for approximately 5 to 7 minutes or until the cabbage is completely wilted. Season liberally with salt and pepper.

6. During this time fry your eggs in a separate pan. Set aside until ready to serve.

7. To serve, top the hash with the cabbage and top the cabbage with the fried eggs.

Pear Pancakes

You can substitute apples for pears and/or all-purpose flour for whole wheat in this recipe and it will still come out plenty delicious! If you don't have buttermilk, use 2 cups of milk with 1 teaspoon of vinegar added. Top with whatever you prefer—if you have any caramel sauce these pancakes basically beg for it.

MAKES APPROXIMATELY 8 MEDIUM PANCAKES

4 tablespoons butter, divided

3 firm pears, spiralized on blade 2

2 cups whole wheat flour

½ teaspoon salt

1 teaspoon baking soda

2 tablespoons brown sugar

2 eggs

2 cups buttermilk

1. In a large skillet, melt 1 tablespoon of butter on medium-high heat.

2. Add the spiralized pears and cook, stirring occasionally until they are softened, about 3 to 4 minutes.

3. Remove the pears and set aside.

4. Combine the flour, salt, baking soda, and brown sugar in a large bowl.

5. In a small bowl, beat the eggs and add the buttermilk. Melt 2 more tablespoons of butter and add it to the eggs and buttermilk. Stir until combined.

6. Add the wet ingredients to the dry and stir until everything is *almost* completely mixed.

7. Using a large spatula, fold the pears gently into the batter.

8. Melt the last tablespoon of butter in the skillet on medium-high heat. Using a ladle, spoon out batches of the batter and cook the pancakes until bubbles begin to form. Flip once and cook until golden brown on both sides, about 3 minutes per side.

The **Veggie Spiral Slicer** Cookbook

Mexican-Inspired Sweet Potato Savory Waffles

This is an unexpected dish in two ways. First, it consists of waffles made out of sweet potatoes, and second, they are distinctly savory. I tend to serve this topped with a fried egg, and every now and then when I'm feeling cheeky, I throw in 1 cup of black beans to get some extra protein in the morning. A drizzle of fresh lime juice never hurts either.

MAKES 4 WAFFLES

1 tablespoon vegetable oil

1 medium sweet potato, spiralized on blade 3

½ yellow onion, spiralized on blade 3

1 medium clove garlic, minced

1 teaspoon ground cumin

1 teaspoon kosher salt

¼ teaspoon cayenne pepper

1 egg plus 1 yolk, beaten

1 tablespoon diced chives

sour cream and salsa, to top (optional)

1. Preheat your waffle iron on medium-high.

2. While your iron is heating up, place the vegetable oil in a large skillet on medium-high heat and add the sweet potato and onion noodles. Stir to coat somewhat with the oil, cover, and cook for 10 minutes. The noodles should begin to soften.

3. Remove the noodles from the pan, allowing them to cool slightly. Place the noodles in a large bowl and add the remaining ingredients.

4. Spray your waffle iron with nonstick cooking spray and fill the bottom with the noodle mixture. Cook according to your waffle iron's guide. The waffles are done when the outsides are crisp, but not burnt, and the interior is soft and warmed.

5. Serve topped with sour cream and salsa if you so choose.

Indian Sweet Noodles with Eggs

This dish, which goes by the name Balaleet, traditionally uses vermicelli noodles. The flavor of the sweet potatoes make this variation similar to a sweet latke, but the decidedly Indian flavor profile makes it a special and surprising breakfast. It's especially delicious topped with a dollop of tangy yogurt and extra orange blossom water.

MAKES 6 SERVINGS

1 medium sweet potato, spiralized on blade 3

2 tablespoons sugar

¼ cup unsalted butter (1 stick), divided

¼ teaspoon saffron threads

½ teaspoon ground cardamom

½ teaspoon ground cinnamon

½ teaspoon curry power

¼ teaspoon ground nutmeg

½ teaspoon salt, plus more to taste

½ teaspoon freshly ground black pepper, plus more to taste

½ teaspoon orange blossom water

6 eggs, beaten

1. In a bowl, toss the sweet potato noodles with the sugar.

2. In a medium skillet, melt half of the butter on medium-high heat. Add the saffron, cardamom, cinnamon, curry powder, nutmeg, salt, and pepper. Stir constantly and cook for 1 minute or until the spices begin to release their aroma.

3. Add the sweet potato noodles to the skillet and stir to coat them with the butter and spice mixture. Press the noodles flat into the skillet until you have what resembles one large noodle pancake. Sprinkle this with orange blossom water. Cook, partially covered and without stirring, for about 15 minutes or until the bottom of the pancake is toasted and the pancake holds together.

4. Flip the pancake and cook, uncovered, for another 10 to 15 minutes or until the other side is toasted and golden brown. Transfer to a plate and keep covered while you make the eggs.

The **Veggie Spiral Slicer** Cookbook

5. Place the now-empty skillet back on medium-high heat and melt the rest of the butter. Add the beaten eggs and season with salt and pepper, to taste. Allow this to cook for about 5 minutes or until the eggs have set. Slide the egg cake out of the pan and cut into wedges to serve on top of the sweet potato noodles. Serve hot.

Cheese Grits

Cheese grits are a Southern staple. If you're not going to be topping yours with jam, then you most likely will be mixing them with cheese. In this version we move from the South to the Southwest with some distinctly Latin flavors.

MAKES 4 SERVINGS

2 tablespoons butter

1 medium clove garlic, minced

1 large sweet potato, spiralized on blade 3, then riced

1 teaspoon smoked paprika

pinch of cayenne pepper (optional)

salt and pepper, to taste

¾ cup chicken stock

½ cup cotija or queso fresco cheese

2 tablespoons chopped chives, plus more to garnish

1. In a large skillet, melt the butter on medium-high heat.

2. Add the garlic and stir constantly, cooking until the garlic beings to release its aroma, about 30 seconds.

3. Put the sweet potato, paprika, cayenne, salt, and pepper in the pan and stir to coat with the garlic butter. Cook until the rice has turned a slightly darker color, about 5 minutes.

4. Pour in the chicken stock and simmer until the liquid has cooked off, but the rice is not yet completely "dry," between 10 and 15 minutes.

5. Remove from the heat and stir in the cheese and chives.

6. Serve hot with a sprinkling of extra chives.

Sweet Potato Sausage Breakfast Burritos

I was always aware of breakfast burritos, but they were never really my thing until I visited Austin, Texas, on a food vacation one year. Now I make them frequently, but rarely with a recipe. They're a great way to get rid of vegetable halves or spiralizer leftovers, but if you are looking for a recipe that's a couple of steps above emptying your fridge, here you have it.

MAKES 4 BURRITOS

3 tablespoons vegetable oil, divided

½ medium sweet potato, spiralized on blade 3

¼ cup chopped green bell pepper

½ pound breakfast sausage, crumbled

2 tablespoons maple syrup

1 medium clove garlic, minced

3 large eggs, beaten

4 (8-inch) flour tortillas

¼ cup sharp cheddar cheese, shredded

1. In a large skillet, heat 2 tablespoons of the vegetable oil on medium-high heat. Add the sweet potato noodles, stir to coat the bottom of the noodles with oil, cover, and cook for 5 minutes.

2. Add the bell pepper and breakfast sausage. Stir and cook for 10 minutes, uncovered. Add the maple syrup and garlic and cook for one more minute. Remove this mixture from the heat and set aside in a paper towel–lined bowl.

3. Wipe the skillet clean and heat up the last tablespoon of vegetable oil on medium heat.

4. Add the beaten eggs and scramble. Cook the eggs until they are set but not dry, approximately 2 minutes. Remove the eggs from the heat.

5. To assemble, place some of the sausage and sweet potato filling in each tortilla. Top with some scrambled egg and sharp cheddar. Roll up and allow the residual heat to melt the cheese. Enjoy!

Candied Ginger and Carrot Scones

It never ceases to amaze me how absolutely nutritionally terrible classic carrot cake is, which is exactly why it's so delicious and why I crave it so often. In my attempt to re-create the flavor profile of classic spiced and sweet carrot cake, I came up with this recipe for scones. It's a lovely and hearty way to start any day, or you can just as easily enjoy it with a cup of tea to hold over any ravenous appetites till lunch. If you would like to, you can use reduced fat cream cheese in this recipe.

MAKES 12 TO 16 SCONES

For the scones:

2 cups whole wheat flour

⅓ cup brown sugar

1 teaspoon baking powder

¼ teaspoon baking soda

½ teaspoon salt

1 teaspoon ground cinnamon

½ teaspoon ground ginger

4 tablespoons frozen cream cheese, cut into cubes

4 tablespoons frozen unsalted butter, cut into cubes

⅔ cup buttermilk

1 egg

2 large carrots, spiralized on blade 3

¼ cup crystalized ginger, minced

For the glaze:

½ cup cream cheese, at room temperature

zest and juice of ½ orange

½ cup powdered sugar

chopped, crystalized ginger, for garnish (optional)

1. Preheat the oven to 400°F and place the baking racks on the middle and lower levels of your oven. Line 2 baking trays with parchment paper.

2. In a large bowl, combine the flour, sugar, baking powder, baking soda, salt, and spices. Move this mixture to your food processor.

3. Pulse in the cream cheese and butter until the chunks are the size of peas. Transfer this mixture back to the large bowl.

4. Whisk the buttermilk and egg together. Pour into the large bowl of dry ingredients.

5. Stir lightly, until almost completely combined. Fold in the carrot noodles and crystalized ginger.

6. Using a large ice cream scoop, portion out 12 to 16 scones, depending on the size of your ice cream scoop. Make sure to use two baking trays and put no more than 8 scones per tray. Bake both trays at the same time for approximately 12 to 15 minutes or until the scones have expanded and are golden brown. Allow to cool completely before glazing.

7. While waiting on the scones to cool, prepare the glaze. Using either a stand mixer, hand mixer, or your strongest arm, whisk the orange juice and zest into the cream cheese until they are homogenized. Whisk in the powdered sugar until you have a sweet mixture that is a drizzling consistency. Drizzle this on top of the scones and top with additional chopped crystalized ginger if you so desire.

Apple Fritters

Apple fritters on their own don't need much of an introduction. In this recipe, I add more apples than usual to make them feel a little less sinful. I prefer Pink Lady apples and Fujis, but if you want to have some fun with it, just pick out any firm baking apples and mix and match!

MAKES 8 TO 12 FRITTERS

vegetable oil, enough to fill your pan at least 1½ inches deep, plus 2 teaspoons

1 cup all-purpose flour

2 teaspoons sugar, plus ¼ cup

1¼ teaspoons baking powder

large pinch of salt

½ cup milk

1 egg, beaten

3 apples, spiralized on blade 2

1 tablespoon ground cinnamon

NOTE: If you add too many fritters to the pan at once, it will shock the oil and lower the temperature, which means they will have to spend more time in the oil, leading to a higher chance they'll become a greasy final product. No bueno. Keep that oil hot, but not smoking, or go the extra mile and use an oil or candy thermometer, keeping the temperature at 375°F.

1. Heat the vegetable oil in a large, high-walled pan over medium-high heat. You want to have enough oil to fill the pan at least 1.5 inches deep but not more than 2 inches.

2. In a bowl, mix the flour, 2 teaspoons sugar, baking powder, and salt.

3. In separate bowl, mix the milk, egg, and 2 teaspoons of vegetable oil. Add to the dry ingredients and mix just until almost combined. (Do not overmix!) Fold the apples noodles in with a spatula until they are mixed in, but still retain some of their shape.

4. Use a greased soup spoon to drop large scoops of the batter into the hot oil. Use the back of the spoon to flatten out the dough ball

somewhat. Fry the fritters, flipping once until they are golden brown on each side.

5. Remove the fritters from the oil and rest them briefly on a plate lined with paper towels.

6. While the fritters drain slightly, mix together the cinnamon and the ¼ cup sugar. While the delicious apple dumplings are still warm, toss them in the cinnamon sugar-mixture and serve immediately.

Spanish Omelet

I first discovered this dish in Barcelona, where it is served at all hours from afternoon until after dinner and goes by the name "tortilla." However, being from the States, in my eyes eggs are meant for breakfast (or frying and putting on top of sandwiches). That being said, feel free to enjoy this quick and delicious dish at any time of the day!

MAKES 4 TO 6 SERVINGS

4 tablespoons olive oil, divided

1 large Russet potato, spiralized on blade 3

6 eggs

2 teaspoons garlic powder

½ teaspoon salt

freshly ground black pepper, to taste

1 medium yellow onion, sliced very thinly

1. In a small skillet, heat 2 tablespoons of the olive oil on medium heat. Make sure to swirl the oil around to cover the bottom of the entire skillet.

2. Place the potato noodles on a plate, cover with a damp paper towel, and microwave for 2 minutes. This will help ensure that the potatoes are cooked all the way through for the finished dish.

3. In a large bowl, stir the eggs, garlic powder, salt, and pepper together. The eggs need to be well blended. Add the onion and potato.

4. Pour the potato and egg mixture into the heated pan. Press the potatoes down so that the top is flattened and the omelet is as compact as possible. Cover and cook on medium heat for approximately 10 minutes.

5. Remove the cover of the skillet and ensure that the omelet has not stuck to the pan by running a large spatula underneath. Gently slide the omelet onto a plate. Add the remaining olive oil to the skillet, keeping the heat on medium-high.

6. Once the oil has heated up, gently slide the Spanish omelet back into the skillet. Cover and cook for another 5 minutes. This helps to brown all sides of the omelet, giving it a nice "set" edge.

7. To serve, place the omelet on a plate, allowing it to cool for a few minutes. Cut into wedges.

Italian-Style Frittata

Simple and flavorful, protein-packed frittatas are an excellent way to add a hearty amount of vegetables into your breakfast. The only requirement is an oven-safe pan. While the frittata sets in the broiler, you can get the orange juice, coffee, side dishes, and/or toast ready.

MAKES 4 TO 6 SERVINGS

1 tablespoon butter

1 medium zucchini, spiralized on blade 3

4 thin slices pancetta, chopped

2 marinated artichoke hearts, roughly chopped

¼ cup mozzarella, chopped into small cubes

6 eggs, beaten

½ teaspoon freshly ground black pepper

1. Preheat your broiler to high.

2. In an oven-safe skillet, melt the butter on medium-high heat. Add the zucchini noodles. Cover and cook, stirring occasionally until the noodles are soft but not fully cooked through, about 5 minutes. Set the noodles aside.

3. Wipe the skillet clean and dry with a paper or kitchen towel. Return the pan to the stove, lower the heat to medium, and add the pancetta and artichoke hearts. Cook, stirring frequently, until the fat on the pancetta becomes translucent, about 4 to 5 minutes. At this point, add the mozzarella and cook without stirring, just until it begins to melt, about 3 minutes. Add the zucchini noodles.

4. Pour in the eggs and stir well one time, just to mix all the ingredients together. Sprinkle with the black pepper. Cook on medium heat until the bottom of the frittata has set and the top begins to.

5. Move the entire pan into your preheated broiler. Cook until the top of the eggs brown slightly, about 3 to 4 minutes.

6. Remove from the oven and serve warm.

Maple Peanut Butter Apple Power Breakfast Bowl

This recipe is one of my favorites in the entire book. Ever since I was a young child, I have loved apples and peanut butter. This recipe takes this familiar concept and matures it with the addition of omega-3–rich chia seeds and naturally sweet maple syrup. It's a filling dish for sure, even though it only calls for one apple. Be forewarned, however, that the dish gets soggy if not consumed within an hour of preparation.

SERVES 1 AS A MEAL OR 2 AS A HEARTY SNACK

1½ tablespoons maple syrup, any grade of your preference

2 tablespoons peanut butter, chunky or creamy

1 sweet red apple, spiralized on blade 3

½ cup crunchy granola or cereal (like an oat cluster cereal)

2 teaspoons chia seeds

1. In a large bowl, whisk the maple syrup into the peanut butter until the two have combined and made a thick paste.

2. Add the apple noodles and toss until the peanut maple sauce coats the apple noodles. After a few minutes, the apples will begin to release some of their juices, which will loosen up the peanut maple paste.

3. Once the apples have been thoroughly coated with the sweetened peanut butter, add the granola and chia seeds. Serve immediately.

Black Pepper Grits with Strawberry Jam

Depending on whom I am talking to, I may explain grits as "Southern risotto without the rice" or risotto as "Italian grits without the hominy." I like my grits on the sweet side, that is, cooked down till creamy, with butter and nice homemade (store-bought is okay too) jam swirled in.

MAKES 2 TO 4 SERVINGS

1 large parsnip, peeled, spiralized on blade 3, then riced

1 tablespoon olive oil

1 teaspoon salt

½ teaspoon (or more if you like) freshly ground black pepper

1 cup whole or 2% milk

¼ cup unsalted butter

4 tablespoons strawberry jam, to top

1. Preheat the oven to 425°F. Line a baking tray with parchment paper.

2. Spread the parsnip rice over the baking tray and drizzle with the olive oil, salt, and pepper. Toss to make sure the parsnip is lightly coated in oil. Alternatively, you can spray the parsnip with a 100 percent oil–based cooking spray.

3. Roast for approximately 5 to 7 minutes, or until the parsnip shows a hint of golden brown color. This will help to release its natural sweetness.

4. In a medium pot, place 1 cup of water and the milk. Bring this mixture to a simmer.

5. Add the parsnip rice and cover.

6. Simmer for about 20 minutes or until the parsnip falls apart when squeezed between two fingers.

7. Remove the lid. If there is still liquid, continue to cook on medium heat, stirring frequently until the liquid is cooked off.

The **Veggie Spiral Slicer** Cookbook

8. Once the grits are "dry," add the unsalted butter and stir until it has melted.

9. To serve, top each serving with 1 to 2 tablespoons of jam, preferably whole-fruit style, and swirl the jam into the grits.

Zucchini Bread

This bread is wonderful as is, but can also be toasted and topped with your favorite chocolate hazelnut spread for an indulgent breakfast or lighter dessert. If (magically) you don't find yourself finishing the whole loaf in time, you can cut this bread up and make it into an out-of-this-world bread pudding.

MAKES 1 LOAF

2½ cups all-purpose flour

1 teaspoon salt

1 teaspoon ground nutmeg

1 teaspoon ground cinnamon

2 teaspoons baking soda

1 cup sugar

1 cup applesauce or vegetable oil, or a blend of the two

4 eggs, beaten

1 teaspoon vanilla extract

2 medium or 1 very large zucchini, spiralized on blade 3

1 cup chopped hazelnuts

1 cup dark chocolate chips

1. Preheat the oven to 350°F. Spray a standard loaf pan with nonstick cooking spray.

2. In a large bowl, whisk the flour, salt, nutmeg, cinnamon, baking soda, and sugar.

3. In a small bowl, combine the applesauce/oil, eggs, and vanilla extract.

4. Add the egg mixture to the dry ingredients and stir until almost combined.

5. Using a spatula, fold in the zucchini, hazelnuts, and chocolate chips. Pour the batter into the prepared loaf pan. Bake for approximately 1 hour, until the top is golden brown and a knife poked into the center comes out clean. Allow to cool for 5 minutes before removing from the pan. Store wrapped in tin foil to maintain freshness.

CHAPTER TWO
Soups

Everyone loves a good soup, and good soup is even better when you replace heavy pasta noodles with zucchini or other vegetables. Everything from classic Irish stew and chicken noodle to the more exotic *asheh reshteh* and *avgolemono* are here to warm up your soul and fill your tummy.

Asheh Reshteh

I'm not going to lie to you, this stunningly hearty and flavorful Persian soup takes a long time to make and a little advance planning, but it's extremely easy and mostly hands off. It also makes a ton of leftovers that get better with time as all the herbs blend together. I made this soup for dinner the first day that I discovered it at lunch in a Mediterranean restaurant—it's that good.

MAKES 8 SERVINGS

For the soup:

2 tablespoons olive oil

2 large yellow onions, spiralized on blade 3

7 cloves garlic, minced

½ cup dried chickpeas, soaked overnight, drained, and rinsed

¼ cup dried red beans, soaked overnight, drained and rinsed

¼ cup frozen lima beans

1 teaspoon turmeric

8 cups vegetable stock

salt and pepper, to taste

½ cup brown lentils

1 bunch fresh parsley, chopped

1 bunch fresh mint, chopped

¼ bunch fresh dill, chopped

3 bunches green onions (green portion only)

1 bunch spinach, chopped

1 medium zucchini, spiralized on blade 3

For the garnish:

2 tablespoons vegetable oil

1 large red onion, spiralized on blade 3

2 tablespoons dried mint

sour cream

1. In a large soup pot, heat the olive oil on medium. Add the onions and cook, stirring occasionally until they are translucent and soft, about 5 to 7 minutes. Add the garlic, stirring constantly, and cook for another 30 seconds.

2. Add the chickpeas, red beans, lima beans, and turmeric. Sauté for 3 to 5 minutes. Add the vegetable stock and bring to a simmer. Cover partially. Cook on medium heat for 1 hour.

3. Add salt and pepper, to taste, and add the lentils, parsley, mint, dill, and green onions. Cook for ½ hour, partially covered.

4. Toss the spinach into the pot and stir for another 5 minutes, or until the spinach has cooked down in size. Add the zucchini noodles. Cover partially and cook for another ½ hour.

5. Remove the cover and simmer the soup for another ½ hour. The soup should thicken.

6. During this last ½ hour, make the garnish. In a large skillet, heat the vegetable oil on medium. Add the onion and cook until it starts to turn clear. Lower the heat to medium-low and allow the onion to caramelize, stirring frequently. Once the onion starts to turn golden, add the dried mint and turn the heat back up to medium. Cook until the onions are crisp.

7. To serve, top the soup with sour cream and the fried red onions.

Chicken Noodle Soup

While writing this book I started to come down with a cold, so I knew I had to make some soup, and stat. Lo and behold, the cold stayed at bay and I was able to remain in the kitchen, cooking away. I believe that the key to great soup is homemade stock, which honestly is the easiest thing in the world to make—but it does take time. If you want to use store-bought stock, you can, just skip the first part of this recipe. Lastly, I usually remove the breasts from the chicken to use in other recipes.

MAKES 6 TO 8 SERVINGS

1 (3- to 4-pound) chicken

1 medium yellow onion, quartered

1 tablespoon olive oil

1 stalk celery, sliced thin

1 large carrot, sliced thin

1 medium yellow onion, diced

2 cloves garlic, minced

1 bay leaf

salt and pepper, to taste

2 medium zucchinis, spiralized on blade 3

To make the stock:

1. In a large pot, cover the chicken with water until the chicken is submerged in water by 1 inch. Add the quartered onion. Bring the pot to a boil on medium-high heat.

2. Cook the chicken until it has been cooked through entirely. Remove it from the water and set aside to cool. Let the water boil until it has reduced by 75 percent. This can take over an hour. You should end up with 4 cups of golden liquid left. Strain the stock and set the liquid aside.

3. Chop 2 cups worth of the cooked chicken and reserve it to use in the soup.

To make the soup:

1. In the same large pot, heat the olive oil on medium-high. Add the celery, carrot, and diced onion. Cook, stirring occasionally, until the carrot and celery are softened and the onion is translucent. Add the garlic and cook for 30 seconds, stirring constantly.

2. At this stage, you should start to see some brown bits forming on the bottom of the pan. This is excellent as long as they are brown and not black. Once you have a nice collection of browning on the bottom of the pan, add a splash (about a tablespoon) of the chicken stock and stir vigorously until you have scraped off all the brown. Add 2 more cups of the chicken stock and 2 cups of water.

3. Add the bay leaf and 2 cups of cooked chicken meat. Reserve the remaining chicken and stock for other recipes. Bring to a simmer and cook, covered, for 10 minutes. Taste. Add salt and pepper, to taste.

4. Add the zucchini noodles and simmer for another 5 minutes. Remove the bay leaf before serving.

Pork Chop Ramen

Ramen inspires a lot of fanaticism. This recipe is far from traditional, but it does make one heck of a satisfying meal in a short period of time. And, sometimes, that's all I need—an awesome, healthy, and delicious meal that I can make more quickly than the time it takes to call and wait for a delivery.

MAKES 4 SERVINGS

2 eggs

2 tablespoons sesame oil

2 boneless pork chops

½ cup soy sauce

½ yellow onion, chopped (about 1 cup)

1 cup sliced button mushrooms

2 cloves garlic, minced

4 cups beef stock

1 zucchini, spiralized on blade 3

1 cup corn kernels

1 sheet toasted nori, cut into thin strips

2 green onions, sliced

1. To hard-boil the eggs, bring a small pot of water to a boil. Add the eggs and cook for 7 minutes. Rinse under water and place in a bowl full of ice water for at least 5 minutes.

2. In a large pot, heat the sesame oil on medium-high. Add the pork chops and cook until each side has begun to brown, about 3 to 4 minutes per side. Splash with the soy sauce halfway through.

3. Add the onion and mushrooms and cook for another 5 minutes. Add the garlic and cook, stirring constantly for 30 seconds.

4. Add the beef stock and bring to a simmer.

5. Add the zucchini noodles and return to a simmer. Cook for 5 minutes.

6. Peel the eggs and slice in half, being careful not to lose any of the yolk, which should be soft and undercooked.

7. Remove the pork chops from the pot and slice thinly.

8. To plate, serve noodles and broth topped with corn, sliced pork chop, halved eggs, nori strips, and sliced green onion.

Pho Bo

Pho *is Vietnam's most famous dish. The warmth and exotic flavor brought by the wealth of spices used in this soup is unparalleled. This soup does take about an hour to make, but most of that time is completely hands off and it will make your kitchen and home smell irresistible.*

MAKES 4 SERVINGS

6 cups beef broth

1 tablespoon ginger, peeled and sliced

2 cinnamon sticks

1 teaspoon black peppercorns, cracked

4 cloves

1 tablespoon coriander seeds

2 tablespoons fish sauce

2 tablespoons brown sugar

2 tablespoons lime juice

1 beef fillet steak, thinly sliced

6 star anise pods

1 large daikon, spiralized on blade 3

2 cups bean sprouts

3 green onions, trimmed, thinly sliced diagonally

1 serrano chile, thinly sliced

½ cup basil leaves, torn

½ cup cilantro leaves, torn

4 to 6 lime wedges, to serve

1. In a large pot, bring the beef broth, ginger, cinnamon, black peppercorns, cloves, coriander seeds, fish sauce, brown sugar, lime juice, and beef fillet to a boil. Simmer, covered, for 45 minutes. Remove the beef fillet and slice it thinly.

2. Add the star anise and simmer for another 5 minutes. Strain all of the spices out of the liquid and return the liquid to the pot. Bring the stock back up to a simmer and add the daikon noodles and beef strips. Cook for another 10 minutes, uncovered.

3. To serve, divvy up the broth and noodles into bowls. Top each serving with the bean sprouts, green onions, sliced chile, basil, cilantro, and 1 lime wedge. Enjoy immediately.

Irish Stew

One of the greatest things about cooking is food's magical ability to take you to faraway lands, even ones you have never been to before. As I write this book, it is a dark and gray 22 degrees outside, but this doesn't mean I don't have to keep training for the strenuous Ireland hiking trip I have planned 6 months from now. That's where this stew comes in, hearty enough to comfort those winter blues, Irish enough to keep me enthralled with dreams of globe-trotting, yet lean enough to help me reach my goals (using portion control, of course.) This meal will feed a small army, a family of four with growing children, or anyone who likes lots of leftovers!

MAKES 6 TO 8 SERVINGS

6 slices thick-cut smoked bacon, roughly chopped

2 pounds lamb stew meat, boneless and cut into chunks

4 large carrots, sliced into rounds

2 large yellow onions, chopped

1 quart lamb, veal, or beef stock

8 sprigs thyme

2 bay leaves

1 teaspoon Worcestershire sauce

1 cup frozen peas

4 medium red potatoes, spiralized on blade 2

NOTE: There are two ways of making this dish: stovetop and slow cooker. I personally prefer the freedom the slow cooker allows. I am able to start this dish then go about my day, adding the spiralized noodles and peas in the last 30 minutes of cooking. If you'd prefer to skip working in the morning and don't mind waiting about 2 hours for everything to be ready from start to finish, then feel free to cook this on your stovetop in a Dutch oven or heavy-bottom pot with a lid covered on medium-low.

1. In a large pan, cook the bacon until it begins to crisp. Add it to your slow cooker. If you are using the stovetop method, cook the bacon in your Dutch oven and set it aside.

2. Brown the lamb in the residual grease from the bacon. It's not a lot of fat but it adds a ton of flavor! Make sure to stir the lamb from time to time so that all the sides are browned, about 5 to 6 minutes. If you are using your slow cooker, add the browned lamb to the cooker, otherwise leave the lamb in the Dutch oven and return the bacon to the pan.

3. Add all of the remaining ingredients, except for the peas and potatoes. For slow cookers, cook this on low for 7 hours. For the Dutch oven, bring the stew to a gentle boil, cover, and lower the heat to medium-low. Allow to cook, covered, for about 90 minutes.

4. Thirty minutes before you want to eat your stew, add the peas and potato noodles. Turn the slow cooker on high or bring your Dutch oven to a simmer on medium-high heat. Cook until the potato noodles are soft and serve, discarding the thyme stems and bay leaves.

Avgolemono

Avgolemono is the classic lemony Greek chicken and rice/orzo soup. It owes its thick and creamy texture to the use of eggs that are beaten quickly. Although this is in no way traditional, I like to add a hearty helping of chopped kale to my batch.

Traditionally, avgolemono is the name for an egg and lemon sauce that you can add to many things (not least of which is chicken soup). It is often made over the course of three hours, starting with a whole chicken. With this recipe, however, soup's on in less than half an hour.

MAKES 4 SERVINGS

4 cups of chicken stock

1 boneless, skinless chicken breast, cubed

1 large or 2 medium parsnips, spiralized on blade 3

2 large eggs

3 teaspoons fresh lemon juice, plus more to serve (optional)

salt and freshly ground black pepper, to taste

3 cups chopped kale (optional)

1. In a large pot, heat the chicken stock and cubed chicken breast. Bring to a boil on medium-high heat, cover, and turn down the heat to medium.

2. Using a food processor, briefly chop the parsnip noodles until they resemble large pieces of rice, or more aptly, orzo. Add the parsnip rice to the pot and cook for approximately 10 minutes, or until the rice begins to soften and the chicken is almost fully cooked through.

3. In a medium bowl, whisk the eggs. Slowly pour in the lemon juice while whisking constantly. Take 1 cup of the chicken stock and very carefully drizzle it into the eggs, all while whisking. Once these have mixed completely, slowly pour the eggs into the soup while stirring vigorously. If you do not keep things moving when combining the eggs and hot liquid, you will end up with scrambled egg soup, which I

can tell you from experience is not a pleasant flavor. If you are using the kale, add it now.

4. Cook while stirring gently on medium heat, uncovered, for 5 minutes or until the soup has thickened, the parsnips are soft, and the kale is wilted. Add your salt and pepper, to taste.

5. Serve topped with a little fresh cracked black pepper and extra lemon if you so desire.

Minestrone

Minestrone soup is such a classic that you can find countless variations. Feel free to play around with this pasta or rice soup served with lots of vegetables and beans, substituting your favorite herbs for the ones listed. Like things hot? Add more red pepper flakes. Above all, have fun!

MAKES 4 TO 6 SERVINGS

2 tablespoons olive oil

1 large carrot, spiralized on blade 3

1 large yellow onion, spiralized on blade 3

1 stalk celery, diced

4 cloves garlic, minced

¼ teaspoon red pepper flakes

1 (14-ounce) can crushed tomatoes

1 (28-ounce) can diced tomatoes, with juice

¼ pound green beans, trimmed and cut to 1-inch pieces

salt and pepper, to taste

1 teaspoon dried oregano

1 teaspoon dried basil

4 cups low-sodium vegetable broth

1 large zucchini, spiralized on blade 1

1 (15-ounce) can cannellini beans

¼ cup grated Parmesan cheese

1. Heat the olive oil in a large pot on medium. Add the carrot, onion, and celery stalk. Sweat the vegetables (cook without browning) until the onions are translucent, about 7 minutes.

2. Add the garlic and red pepper flakes and cook, stirring constantly, for 30 seconds.

3. Add both types of tomatoes to the pot and stir to combine. Cook for another minute.

4. Add the green beans, salt, pepper, oregano, basil, and vegetable broth. Bring to a boil. Reduce the heat to a simmer, cover, and cook for 10 minutes.

5. Once the 10 minutes have passed, uncover, add the zucchini noodles and cannellini beans, and cook for another 5 minutes or until the noodles are softened.

6. Serve topped with grated Parmesan.

Mexican Noodle Soup (Sopa de Fideo)

I love using crisped potato noodles in place of al dente vermicelli. They bring a nice toasty and earthy flavor to the party that is both instantly familiar and unexpected. This acidic and light soup is a great start to any Mexican-themed meal, but I also love it as a light lunch on hot days.

MAKES 4 SERVINGS

¼ cup vegetable oil, divided

2 stalks celery, diced

2 large carrots, spiralized on blade 3

1 yellow onion, spiralized on blade 3

4 cloves garlic, minced

1 (28-ounce) can diced tomatoes, with juice

1 teaspoon ground cumin

4 cups vegetable or chicken stock

1 Russet potato, spiralized on blade 3 and chopped into 1- to 2-inch noodles

juice of 1 lime

1. In a large pot, heat up 2 tablespoons of the vegetable oil on medium-high.

2. Add the celery, carrots, and onion and cook, stirring occasionally, for 5 to 7 minutes or until the onion is translucent. You do not want to caramelize them.

3. Add the garlic and stir constantly for 30 seconds. Add the tomatoes with juice and cumin. Cook for another 5 minutes.

4. Pour the vegetable or chicken stock into the pot and bring the soup to a boil. Reduce the heat to a simmer, cover, and let cook for 30 minutes.

5. While the soup is cooking, heat the remaining vegetable oil in a large skillet on medium-high. Fry the potato noodles until they are browned and crispy.

6. Add the crunchy potato noodles to the soup during the last 5 minutes of cooking.

7. Sprinkle the lime juice over each individual bowl of soup right before serving and enjoy!

Thai Noodle Soup

The lovely and unmistakable flavors of Thai food really shine through in this soup. Spicy ginger mingles with fresh and bright lemongrass and lime. The hint of sweet brown sugar marries with the hot chili sauce perfectly, and the hearty dark meat chicken stands up to all of the flavors. This dish takes less than 20 minutes to prepare once you have your ingredients at the ready.

MAKES 4 TO 6 SERVINGS

4 cups chicken stock

2 carrots, spiralized on blade 3

1 bunch green onions, sliced thin

2 tablespoons fish sauce

1 tablespoon soy sauce

1 tablespoon Thai hot chili sauce

4 cloves garlic, minced

2 tablespoons ginger, grated fine then measured

1 tablespoon chopped fresh basil

1 tablespoon brown sugar

1 stalk lemongrass, cracked

8 ounces any dark meat chicken, chopped

2 large zucchinis, spiralized on blade 3

2 cups chopped bok choy greens

1 cup button mushrooms, sliced

cilantro, for garnish

juice and zest of 1 lime, for garnish

1. In a large pot, bring the chicken stock plus 4 cups of water to a boil. Add the carrots, green onions, fish sauce, soy sauce, hot chili sauce, garlic, ginger, basil, brown sugar, lemongrass, and chicken. Reduce the heat and simmer for 10 minutes.

2. Add zucchini noodles, boy choy, and mushrooms. Cook for another 5 minutes.

3. Remove lemongrass before serving. Garnish with fresh cilantro, lime zest, and sprinkles of the lime juice on each bowl.

Beet Tarator

Tarator *is the national food of Bulgaria, and for good reason. Traditionally it combines crisp cucumbers with tangy yogurt, fresh dill, savory garlic, and crunchy walnuts, and turns all of that delightfulness into a chilled soup that is absolutely perfect for a hot day. In this recipe, the water that is released from the cucumbers works to your benefit and gives the soup a fresher flavor than just using water alone, so do not pre-salt or drain them. I like to use pecans in place of walnuts and add extra vegetables to the party to make what is usually served as a light starter course into a solid meal. Beets work especially well and make this soup a fun and bright pink.*

MAKES 4 SERVINGS

2 large cucumbers, spiralized on blade 2

2 medium red beets, spiralized on blade 3

3 cups Greek yogurt

4 cloves garlic, minced

¼ cup toasted pecans, chopped, plus extra for topping

1 bunch fresh dill, chopped

1 tablespoon olive oil

1 teaspoon salt

½ teaspoon freshly ground black pepper

1. In a large bowl, stir all of the ingredients together and let rest in the refrigerator for 1 hour, allowing the liquid to come out of the cucumbers.

2. Check the consistency of the soup. If it is too thick to pour, add water ¼ cup at a time. You want this to resemble very chunky and pink pancake batter. It's important not to make this soup too thin.

3. Serve well-chilled and topped with extra pecans.

CHAPTER THREE
Salads

These salads are here to entice you. I eat a salad every day and there is no way I could keep this up if they were boring. Yes, there are some classic green salads in here, but they are all absolutely bursting with flavor, and sometimes the occasional unexpected ingredient. The Great Winter Salad is one of the best recipes in this book, if you ask me. Feeling adventurous? Try the Russian *shuba*, or fish salad—you'll be glad you did. This section also contains a lovely handful of French salads or slaws. So go ahead, get your salad on and your body will thank you.

Great Winter Salad

This recipe has been a favorite of mine since I moved far away from the tropical warmth of Florida to the harsh winters of Chicago and eventually settled down in New York City. This delightful salad is full of flavors, colors, and textures, and thanks to the hemp seeds, it has a decent amount of protein. It's the perfect midwinter breakfast. Or lunch, snack, dessert, or.... Like any recipe that focuses on a select few fresh raw fruits, the quality of the final dish is totally dependent on the quality and ripeness of your pears and persimmons. If your persimmons are not soft and squishy (without being too ripe) their astringent juices will taint the flavor of the rest of the dish. If your pears are not ripe, the consequences are less severe, but you won't experience the full potential of this dish, and I'd just hate to see that happen. In the winter, I recommend having extra persimmons and pears lying around. To quote the amazing pastry chef Emily Luchetti, "You have to have a premeditated use for pears." For this recipe, I prefer to use a Bosc pear, but any pear that you enjoy is fine.

MAKES 1 SERVING AS A MEAL OR 2 AS A SNACK

1 pear, spiralized using blade 3

1 ripe fuyu or hachiya persimmon, cubed small

3 to 4 pitted dates, minced

¼ cup goji berries

3 tablespoons hemp seeds

2 tablespoons honey

dash of ground cinnamon, to taste

1. In a bowl, lightly toss the pear noodles, cubed persimmon, minced dates, goji berries, and hemp seeds.

2. Drizzle the honey over the salad and mix until everything is coated with a light layer of honey. The pear will eventually begin to release some of its juices, and this is fine. I use chopsticks to mix everything without being too rough, but that's a purely personal quirk.

3. Sprinkle with a couple of dashes of cinnamon to your own taste and enjoy!

Anchovy and Escarole Salad

Raw broccoli can have a very strong flavor. Some people love it and others, well, not so much. The same can be said for anchovies, which is why I feel that this recipe works so well. The bitter of the raw ingredients plays with the savory and the sweet of the roasted ones.

MAKES 4 SERVINGS

For the salad:

1 head broccoli, florets cut off and stem spiralized on blade 3

2 cups shaved Brussels sprouts

¾ cup extra virgin olive oil, divided

salt and pepper, to taste

For the dressing:

3 anchovy fillets, drained and chopped coarsely

2 cloves garlic, chopped

2 egg yolks

¼ cup chopped parsley

2 tablespoons lemon juice

2 medium heads of escarole, green and yellow leaves only, torn into large pieces

½ cup freshly grated Pecorino Romano cheese

1. Preheat the oven to 450°F.

2. Line 2 baking trays with parchment paper. Toss the broccoli florets (reserve the broccoli noodles for later) and shaved Brussels sprouts with 2 tablespoons of the olive oil. Season liberally with salt and pepper. Roast for approximately 15 minutes or until the florets and sprouts begin to get some color to them. Allow them to cool completely.

3. While the sprouts are roasting, blend the anchovies, garlic, egg yolks, parsley, and lemon juice in either a high-speed blender or food processor to make your dressing. Once you have reached a paste-like consistency, slowly add the remaining olive oil from the salad ingredients until it is emulsified.

4. To make the salad, toss the raw broccoli noodles, roasted broccoli florets and Brussels sprouts, dressing, escarole pieces, and cheese together until everything is coated in the dressing. Serve chilled or at room temperature.

Shuba

Shuba means "fur coat" in Russian, and this salad is referred to as "herring in a fur coat" because of the way it's traditionally presented and layered. My taste buds prefer smoked salmon, but you can substitute the original herring fillets in its place and the dish will still come out great. The vegetables are usually boiled and grated, but I prefer to roast them just until softened and toss the whole batch together.

MAKES 6 TO 8 SERVINGS

4 tablespoons olive oil

6 small red new potatoes, spiralized on blade 3

3 medium red beets, spiralized on blade 2

4 medium carrots, spiralized on blade 3

4 eggs

1 pound smoked salmon, chopped

1 small red onion, diced

2 cups mayonnaise

2 cups chopped fresh spinach

4 sprigs dill, chopped

1. Preheat the oven to 450°F and line 3 baking trays with parchment paper.

2. In a large bowl, toss the potatoes with the olive oil and place them on one of the baking trays. Repeat this with the carrots and the beets. Make sure not to crowd the baking trays. Roast the potatoes in the oven for 15 to 20 minutes or until they are soft. The beets will most likely be ready between 10 to 15 minutes so you may want to pull them out early. The carrots will need about 15 minutes. Set the vegetables aside and allow them to cool completely before using.

3. In the meantime, hard-boil the eggs. Bring a medium pot of water to a boil. Add the eggs, cover, and turn off the heat. Allow the eggs to sit in the water for 10 minutes before running them under cold water until they are cool to the touch. Allow the eggs to cool completely before using. Peel, then using a cheese grater, grate the eggs and set aside.

4. Toss the vegetable noodles, eggs, salmon, red onion, mayonnaise, spinach, and dill in a large bowl. Allow this to chill in the refrigerator for at least 30 minutes before serving.

Greek Salad

Unless you are in an actual Greek restaurant, most of the Greek salads you will see on menus are nothing more than lettuce, cucumbers, olives, and feta cheese. Horiatiki salads, or village salads, are the true authentic Hellenic way to go, not this iceberg lettuce nonsense. This Horiatiki classic dish takes less than 10 minutes to prep, but it does benefit from a half-hour rest in the refrigerator before serving, to let the vinaigrette take the edge off of the raw red onions.

MAKES 2 SERVINGS AS A LARGE SALAD OR 4 AS A SIDE SALAD

1 large cucumber, spiralized on blade 2

1 medium tomato, cut into small wedges

½ green bell pepper, cut into thin strips

½ red onion, sliced into thin strips

¼ to ½ pound feta cheese, crumbled

¾ cup kalamata olives, pitted

½ cup extra virgin olive oil

¼ cup red wine vinegar

2 teaspoons sea salt

2 teaspoons dried oregano

1. In a large bowl, combine the cucumber, tomato, bell pepper, onion, feta, and olives.

2. Drizzle the olive oil and red wine vinegar over the salad. Toss to mix. Allow to rest in the refrigerator for 30 minutes before tossing again and topping with the sea salt and oregano right before serving.

Beet Apple Salad

Beets, apples, and gorgonzola go together perfectly in this bright pink salad. It may seem like an annoyance to swap the spiralizer blade for the apples, but being cut larger gives them the extra crunch they need to hold up to the deep flavor of the beets and cheese.

MAKES 4 SERVINGS

For the salad:

1 pound red beets, spiralized on blade 3

salt and pepper, to taste

2 Fuji, Pink Lady, or other sweet apple, spiralized on blade 2

½ cup crumbled gorgonzola

½ cup toasted hazelnuts, chopped

For the dressing:

½ cup apple cider vinegar

3 tablespoons honey

½ teaspoon kosher salt

¼ cup plus 2 tablespoons extra virgin olive oil

1. Preheat the oven to 425°F and line 2 baking trays with parchment paper. Spread the spiralized beets on the trays and sprinkle liberally with salt and pepper. Roast for 5 to 7 minutes or until the beets are softened.

2. Allow the beets to cool completely. In a large bowl, mix the beet noodles, apple noodles, gorgonzola, and hazelnuts.

3. To make the dressing, whisk the vinegar, honey, and salt. Slowly whisk in the olive oil until the dressing is homogenized.

4. Pour the dressing over the salad, toss, and allow to rest for 5 minutes before serving.

Roasted Beet and Goat Cheese Salad

Caraway is one of those ingredients that always seems terribly underrated. It ranks right up there with beets in unique and earthy deliciousness, and both deserve spots in your kitchen. On top of that, both of these flavors blend together wonderfully well.

MAKES 2 SERVINGS AS A LARGE SALAD OR 4 AS A SIDE SALAD

For the salad:

1 pound red beets, spiralized on blade 3

salt and pepper, to taste

¼ cup crumbled goat cheese

1 green onion, sliced thinly

For the dressing:

¼ cup walnut oil

¼ cup whole-grain mustard

¼ cup red wine vinegar

1 tablespoon caraway seeds

1. Preheat the oven to 425°F and line 2 baking trays with parchment paper. Spread the spiralized beets on the trays and sprinkle liberally with salt and pepper. Roast for 5 to 7 minutes or until the beets are softened.

2. Allow the beets to cool completely. In a large bowl, mix the beet noodles, goat cheese, and green onion.

3. To make the dressing, mix the walnut oil, mustard, vinegar, and caraway seeds in a small bowl. Drizzle over the beets and toss gently to combine.

Great Grandma Dorothy's Marinated Salad

For some reason or another, my family has passed down only a handful of recipes, but the select few are wonderful. This recipe makes a large amount and it's ridiculously delicious. It comes to you courtesy of my Great Grandmother Dorothy. The dressing will need to be shaken before use, as the vinegar and oil separate and the pimentos sink to the bottom.

SALAD MAKES 4 SERVINGS, SALAD DRESSING MAKES EXTRA

For the salad:

2 large carrots, spiralized on blade 3

1 medium red beet, spiralized on blade 3

1 medium red onion, spiralized on blade 3

1 small jicama, spiralized on blade 3

3 cups iceberg lettuce

½ cup shredded cheddar cheese (optional)

For Great Grandma Dorothy's salad dressing:

2 cups sugar

2 cups red wine vinegar

2 tablespoons Worcestershire sauce

½ cup neutral vegetable oil

1 large yellow onion, diced

2 tablespoons kosher salt

1 (4-ounce) jar pimentos, drained

1. To make the salad, toss all of ingredients in a large bowl.

2. To make the dressing, combine all of the ingredients in a large jar with a lid and shake until the sugar dissolves.

3. Drizzle your preferred amount of the dressing over the salad and enjoy!

Broccoli Salad

The sheer amount of raw broccoli in this recipe helps to counter the fact that it contains both sugar and mayonnaise. Feel free to substitute lighter versions of the mayo and yogurt if you so choose, but if you do, you may want to decrease the amount of sugar you use, as many low-fat versions of foods have added sugars in them. This is a great picnic or barbecue recipe.

MAKES 4 SERVINGS

For the salad:

1 large head broccoli, with the long stem intact

1 carrot, spiralized on blade 3, then riced

½ cup red onion, diced

½ cup golden raisins

½ cup sunflower seeds

½ cup chopped red bell pepper

For the dressing:

½ cup mayonnaise

½ cup Greek yogurt

2 tablespoons red wine vinegar

2 tablespoons sugar

salt and pepper, to taste

1. Carefully cut the broccoli florets off of the stem, making sure to leave the stem whole.

2. Spiral slice the stem on blade 3.

3. Combine the broccoli, carrot, red onion, raisins, sunflower seeds, and bell pepper in a large bowl.

4. To make the dressing, mix the mayonnaise, Greek yogurt, red wine vinegar, sugar, salt, and pepper in a small bowl.

5. Add the dressing to the broccoli mix and stir until everything is combined.

6. Allow the salad to rest in the refrigerator for at least 30 minutes before serving to ensure that it is well-chilled.

Carrot Salad

After spending quite a bit of time in France, I got accustomed to the vinegar-dressed carrot slaws that could be found ready packed in all the grocery stores. The dish is not unlike something you would find in a big city deli, only more, well, French.

MAKES 4 SERVINGS

For the salad:

¼ cup raisins

¼ cup walnuts, chopped

2 tablespoons chopped tarragon

1 ½ pounds carrots, spiralized on blade 3

zest of 1 small orange

For the dressing:

2 tablespoons walnut oil

3 tablespoons whole-grain Dijon mustard

2 tablespoons apple cider vinegar

1. In a large bowl, mix the raisins, walnuts, tarragon, carrot noodles, and orange zest. Toss to combine.

2. To make the dressing, in a small bowl, whisk the walnut oil into the Dijon mustard. Continue to whisk and add the cider vinegar.

3. Add the dressing to the salad, mix to coat the salad entirely, and refrigerate for 30 minutes to marinate before serving.

Pear Cucumber Salad

This is the kind of salad I like to pair with any kind of Asian soup–based dish like ramen, bibimbap, or pho. It's also a wonder the next day in a packed lunch, unlike the leafy green salads that are prone to wilting. Any salad that can survive as leftovers is a winner in my book.

MAKES 2 SERVINGS

1 D'Anjou pear, spiralized on blade 2

½ medium cucumber, spiralized on blade 2

2 teaspoons sesame oil

2 tablespoons toasted sesame seeds

3 tablespoons rice wine vinegar

1 tablespoon soy sauce

2 tablespoons honey

2 sheets toasted nori, cut into thin strips

1. Combine all ingredients in a large bowl. Toss to coat. Chill in the refrigerator for 30 minutes, stirring once halfway through, and once right before serving. Enjoy!

Fennel Apple Salad

Salads are my favorite way to do lunch. They are quick and easy and leave you feeling satisfied without being weighed down. Feel free to substitute any nuts or dried fruits that you prefer. This dish also works with Meyer lemons in place of the oranges; you will need two Meyer lemons to equal one orange.

MAKES 2 SERVINGS AS A MEAL OR 4 AS A SIDE SALAD

For the salad:

1 medium fennel bulb, spiralized on blade 3

1 apple, any sweet red variety, spiralized on blade 3

½ red onion, sliced thin

3 cups arugula

½ cup grated Parmesan cheese

¼ cup chopped toasted almonds

¼ cup Thompson raisins

For the dressing:

juice and zest of 1 orange

¼ cup extra virgin olive oil

1 tablespoon Dijon mustard

⅛ teaspoon salt

1. In a large bowl combine all of the salad ingredients.

2. In a small bowl, whisk the dressing ingredients together.

3. Drizzle the dressing over the salad and toss to combine.

Tuna Salad

This salad came about one night when I was too tired to cook. It has now become a staple in my fridge for its flexibility as a side dish and sandwich filler, and the fact that it makes a great pre-workout snack stuffed into a lettuce leaf.

MAKES 4 SERVINGS

For the salad:

1 medium zucchini

2 (5-ounce) cans water-packed tuna, drained and flaked

½ red onion, chopped fine

½ green bell pepper, chopped fine

For the horseradish mix:

2 teaspoons grated fresh horseradish

2 tablespoons Dijon mustard

½ cup sour cream

1 teaspoon garlic powder

salt and pepper, to taste

1. Slice the zucchini lengthwise halfway to the middle. Make sure you do not cut the zucchini in half! Using blade 1, spiral slice the zucchini so that you have short, curled pieces. Place these in a large bowl. You can skip the salting and squeezing step here.

2. In a medium bowl, add the tuna, onion, and green pepper to your zucchini noodles. Stir to mix everything.

3. In a small bowl, mix the horseradish, Dijon mustard, sour cream, garlic powder, salt, and pepper.

4. Pour the horseradish mix onto the salad and stir to combine.

5. Chill in the refrigerator for at least 30 minutes. Serve chilled.

Golden Beet with Blood Orange and Miso Salad

This salad is one of my favorites to take on summer picnics. In order to make it "to go," I merely wait to add the spinach until the moment I am going to serve it. This salad is especially delicious served chilled, directly from the refrigerator. The lovely amount of color is sure to brighten anyone's day!

MAKES 2 SERVINGS

For the salad:

2 golden beets, spiralized on blade 3

salt and pepper, to taste

3 cups baby spinach

2 green onions, sliced thin

For the dressing:

2 tablespoons white miso

1/3 cup fresh orange juice

2 tablespoons extra virgin olive oil

1 shallot, minced

1 blood orange, segmented and chopped

1. Preheat the oven to 425°F. Line a baking tray with parchment paper. Spread the beet noodles evenly on the tray, using a second tray if necessary. Sprinkle lightly with salt and pepper. Roast in the oven for approximately 5 minutes, or until the color of the beets deepens and the noodles become soft. Once the beets are cooled, toss with the baby spinach and green onions in a large bowl.

2. To make the dressing, mix the white miso and orange juice, making sure there are no clumps of miso left over. Stir in the olive oil, shallot, and orange segments.

3. Drizzle the dressing on top of the salad and enjoy!

Potato and Green Bean Salad

At this point, I am beginning to feel like this book should have a "vegetable salads inspired by France" section. But all joking aside, the French do know what to do with their veggies. Usually it involves slathering them in Dijon and vinegar, and I am more than okay with that.

MAKES 4 TO 6 SERVINGS

4 large eggs

1 pound green beans, trimmed and cut to 1-inch lengths

⅓ cup plus 2 tablespoons extra virgin olive oil

2 pounds medium yellow potatoes, like Yukon Gold, spiralized on blade 3

salt and pepper, to taste

1 large thyme sprig

3 cloves garlic, minced fine

1 tablespoon chopped capers

2 teaspoons Dijon mustard

4 tablespoons white wine vinegar

2 tablespoons thinly sliced chives

2 tablespoons roughly chopped parsley

8 ounces baby spinach, chopped

1. To hard-boil the eggs, bring a large pot of salted water to a boil. Add the eggs, turn off the heat, cover, and allow the eggs to sit for 12 minutes. Remove the eggs and rinse them under cold water. Place the eggs in an ice water bath.

2. Bring the water back to a boil. Cook the green beans for 5 minutes. Drain the beans and run them under cold water to stop the cooking and chill the beans.

3. In a large skillet on medium-high heat, add the 2 tablespoons of olive oil. Add the potato noodles, salt, pepper, and thyme. Stir to coat, cover, and cook, stirring occasionally for 5 to 7 minutes or until the potato noodles are cooked through. Set aside to cool.

4. While the potato noodles are cooking, peel the eggs. Cut them into quarter wedges and set aside.

5. Mix the dressing. In a large bowl, whisk the garlic, salt, pepper, chopped capers, Dijon mustard, and white wine vinegar. Once that is all combined, whisk in the remaining olive oil. Add the cut eggs, green beans, potato noodles, chives, parsley, and chopped baby spinach.

6. Allow to sit in the refrigerator until the spinach begins to wilt, at least 20 minutes.

7. Serve cold or at room temperature.

CHAPTER FOUR
Sides

This is the fun wildcard section, where you'll find everything from appetizers to dips to roasted veggies. Learn how to save time making the classic latke, what dip is good to have on hand to dress up salads and sandwiches, how to make a couple of quick pickles, and what to do with all those mushroom-shaped pieces your spiral slicer leaves behind. This section is like the A-Team of spiral-sliced recipes. Each one is unique, awesome, and ready to kick some butt (or at least rock your taste buds). What are you waiting for?

Red Pepper Sun-Dried Tomato Dip

I love the versatility of dips. Having this roasted red pepper spread in the refrigerator means that at any time, you can dress up basic sandwiches, have a light snack with some raw veggies, or thin it out and mix in some hearty kale to make a well-dressed salad full of protein, vitamins, and flavor! Serve with toasted pita, chips, crudités, or as a spread on sandwiches.

MAKES APPROXIMATELY 2½ CUPS

½ cup sun-dried tomatoes, not packed in oil

1 roasted red bell pepper

1 large clove garlic

1 (15-ounce) can cannellini beans, rinsed and drained

1 teaspoon salt

¼ to ½ cup olive oil

1 cucumber, spiralized on blade 3

1. In a food processor, blend the sun-dried tomatoes, roasted red pepper, garlic clove, cannellini beans, and salt until a smooth paste forms. Slowly add the ¼ cup olive oil while running the food processor. If your pepper spread is still too thick, slowly add the remaining olive oil until you achieve a smooth paste.

2. Combine the pepper paste and spiralized cucumber in a bowl and serve.

Latkes

Latkes were one of the first recipes I made with a spiralizer. Everyone loves latkes, but I have yet to meet anyone who loves shredding the potatoes to make them. The spiralizer makes quick work of the classic spud, and you're that much closer to fried potato cake bliss. In fact, why are you still reading this? Latkes await!

Personally, I enjoy my latkes pretty straightforward—a nice mix of potato and onion—but feel free to add any herbs or cheeses that you fancy. For this recipe, a scant tablespoon of minced, fresh herbs and anywhere from ¼ to ½ cup of shredded cheese can be added into the mix right before frying. Serve with sour cream, applesauce, Greek yogurt, a fried egg, pork chops, the list goes on...

MAKES 4 TO 6 SERVINGS

vegetable oil for frying, enough to fill your pan ½ inch deep with oil

2 medium potatoes, preferably Russet or Yukon Gold, spiralized on blade 3

1 medium yellow onion, diced fine

1 clove garlic, minced

2 eggs, beaten

1 teaspoon baking powder

salt and pepper, to taste

1. Fill a large frying pan with vegetable oil until it's about ½ inch deep. Heat the oil on medium-high.

2. While the oil is heating up, wrap the potato noodles in paper towels and microwave for 2 minutes. Press the noodles to drain of any excess liquid afterward.

3. Mix the potatoes with the onion, garlic, eggs, baking powder, salt, and pepper.

4. Test the oil to see if it's hot enough. I do this by adding the smallest piece of potato noodle and watching to see if it instantly sizzles. Once the oil is ready, add the potato noodles in small batches to the pan. Use a spatula to press them flat, creating a small pancake shape.

Add more noodles and work in small batches, making sure not to overcrowd the pan. If the heat begins to dip, wait on adding your next batch until your oil temperature has risen once more. If you add your latkes to oil that is not hot enough, you will end up with soggy latkes, and those are not what we want. Flip the latkes one time and cook until the delicious little pancake is golden brown on both sides, about 3 to 4 minutes per side.

5. Remove from the oil and rest on a paper towel–lined plate.

6. Serve warm.

Curly Fries Two Ways

Truly there are two different types of curly fries: the classic slinky-style potato type that most of us have encountered in the grocery store freezer section or at certain fast-food joints and the shoestring style that you've seen either compressed into hash browns or bought fried crisp and packaged in a can, shelf stable as can be. I'm not one to knock convenience; in fact, I find the convenience of the spiralizer to be one of its biggest selling points. But I always prefer to enjoy fresh homemade fries as opposed to ones out of a drive-through window or a can. These fries could more realistically be called "bakes," but they are healthier and less prone to falling apart or making an oily mess.

MAKES 4 SERVINGS

2 large potatoes, sweet potatoes, or parsnips, spiralized on blade 2 for curly fries, on blade 3 for shoestring fries

3 tablespoons olive oil

kosher salt and pepper, to taste

NOTE: It's very important not to crowd your baking sheet. The fries won't crisp up properly if you do. Either use a second tray or work in batches.

1. Preheat the oven to 400°F and position your baking racks as close to the middle as possible.

2. In a large bowl, use your hands to combine the spiralized fries and olive oil until all the vegetables are well coated.

3. Spread the fries out evenly on parchment paper–coated baking trays. (Parchment works much better than tin foil and is not going to tear when you stir the fries mid-cooking.) Sprinkle with salt and pepper.

4. Bake on the middle oven rack for approximately 30 minutes for shoestring fries and 40 to 45 minutes for curly fries. Every 15 minutes or so, check and stir your fries to prevent sticking and burning.

Variations: Feel free to add some seasonings. I enjoy steak seasonings on my potato fries and a mixture of ¼ cup brown sugar and ½ teaspoon of cayenne pepper on my sweet potatoes. To add these seasonings evenly, I gently massage them into the fries during the oiling process.

Spring Rolls

Spring rolls were one of the first applications I thought of when I was intro-duced to the spiral slicer. The light and fresh rice wrappers are a wonderful vehicle for all kinds of fruits and veggies, and the slicer does a great job of quickly chopping up fillings. Feel free to branch off of the traditional styles and stuff yours with cooked sweet potato noodles and peppers or whatever you prefer! Just make sure not to overstuff the fragile wrappers.

MAKES 8

8 large (8½-inch diameter) rice wrappers

1 zucchini, spiralized on blade 3

1 carrot, spiralized on blade 3

2 cups jicama, spiralized on blade 3

1 mango, peeled and cut into long strips

8 large precooked shrimp, peeled, deveined, and cut in half

2 tablespoons chopped fresh basil leaves

2 tablespoons chopped fresh mint leaves

2 tablespoons chopped fresh cilantro leaves

3 green onions, sliced thin

hoisin sauce, to serve

1. Set up your rolling station with a clean kitchen towel, a plate, and a bowl full of warm water laid out. Lay out your wrappers, spiralized vegetables, mango, and shrimp.

2. In a small bowl, mix the fresh herbs and green onions. Place with the remaining ingredients.

3. Quickly dunk one of the rice wrappers in the warm water to soften it. Lay it flat on the kitchen towel. Place a split shrimp in the middle of the wrapper and top with the spiralized veggies, allowing for 2 inches of free space on each of the four sides of the vegetable fillings. Sprinkle on some of the fresh herb mix.

4. To roll, fold in the top 2-inch flap and then the bottom 2 inches of wrapper. Fold over the right side of the open flap. Starting from the left tightly roll closed the last uncovered side.

5. Repeat with the remaining wrappers and ingredients.

6. Serve with hoisin sauce, chilled or at room temperature.

Tzatziki

There's a lot of talk among food professionals about what their death row last meal would be. While this sounds morbid, it's more of a positive discussion, as any who have been privy to one of these exchanges could easily witness. Eyes glaze over in rapt recollection of mom's potato gratin, perfectly seared fillets, and even peanut butter and jelly sandwiches. Without hesitation, my death row meal would be a bowl of tzatziki sauce big enough to dive into, served with a mountain of lightly toasted pita bread drizzled in olive oil and sprinkled with minuscule boulders of crunchy sea salt.

Tzatziki is one of the simplest recipes to make, but nothing makes it taste better than letting it age in the fridge for an evening. If you skip the resting stage it will still be delicious, but resting spells the difference between a really good dish and a really great one.

MAKES APPROXIMATELY 2½ CUPS

1 large seedless cucumber, spiralized on blade 2

4 teaspoons kosher or sea salt, divided

2 cups Greek yogurt

4 cloves garlic, minced

1½ tablespoons white vinegar

1. Lay 2 paper towels over a pasta strainer in the sink. Add the cucumber noodles and sprinkle with 2 of the teaspoons of salt. Allow the cucumbers to sit for 5 to 10 minutes or until they release most of their water. This step is crucial or you will end up with something closer to soup than sauce.

2. While you wait, mix the Greek yogurt, garlic, remaining salt, and vinegar in a medium bowl.

3. Squeeze out the cucumber noodles, getting as much liquid out of them as possible without breaking them. Add them to the yogurt mixture and fold with a spatula to combine everything.

4. Allow to rest in the refrigerator for one evening. Serve on top of burgers, with pita bread, on salads, basically anywhere. This stuff if pretty darn magical.

Thai Sweet-Pickled Cucumber Salad

Despite the name containing the word "salad," this dish is considered more of a slaw or side and is basically a riff on that small dish of quick-pickled cucumbers that one receives alongside their chicken satay in most Thai restaurants. It's a nice, unexpectedly and distinctly Thai recipe to have on hand, and the cucumbers can last nearly a week in the fridge. The unexpected brightness of the vinegar and sweetness of the sugar make this a light and pleasant topping for chicken sandwiches or cutlets (even without the traditional peanut sauce).

MAKES 4 SERVINGS

½ cup sugar

½ cup rice wine vinegar

1 teaspoon kosher salt

1 cucumber, English is best, spiralized on blade 3

1 small shallot, sliced thinly

1 small Thai chile, seeded and stemmed

NOTE: These should be made at least 4 hours in advance.

1. In a small saucepan, combine the sugar, vinegar, and salt on medium-high heat, stirring constantly. Once the sugar has dissolved and the liquid is warm but not hot, turn off the heat. Place the mixture in the fridge, uncovered, and allow to cool.

2. While the mixture is cooling, mix the cucumber noodles, shallot, and chile in a small nonreactive glass or plastic container with a lid.

3. Once the liquid is cooled, pour the sweetened vinegar over the noodles. Cover, shake to combine well, and allow to rest in the refrigerator for a minimum of 4 hours before serving.

Cheesy Spaghetti Fritters

These are an indulgent treat that work great as a party snack, even if only to prevent you from eating the entire batch yourself! Smoky, salty, creamy, and crunchy, these will satisfy nearly every craving imaginable.

MAKES 6 SERVINGS

4 ounces bacon, cut into ¼-inch pieces

1 large white potato, spiralized on blade 3

8 tablespoons unsalted butter

1 cup all-purpose flour, divided

4 cups heavy cream

8 ounces smoked mozzarella, cut into ¼-inch pieces

salt and pepper, to taste

2 cups panko breadcrumbs

1 teaspoon ground cumin

canola oil, for frying

1. In a large skillet on medium heat, cook the bacon pieces until they are crisp. Remove them from the pan and set aside.

2. While the bacon is cooking, slice the potato lengthwise halfway to the center, taking care not to cut all the way through. Slice the potato on blade 3 of the spiral slicer.

3. Heat the leftover bacon drippings on medium heat and add the potato noodles. Cook until crisped, about 5 to 7 minutes. Set them aside to cool.

4. In a medium pot, melt the butter on medium heat. Stir in ½ cup of the all-purpose flour and continue to stir nonstop for about 2 minutes. The mixture should start to thicken. Pour in the cream, allow this mixture to come to a boil, and lower the heat. Cook, stirring frequently, until the cream reduces some and the liquid thickens, about 5 minutes. Set this aside.

5. In a large bowl, mix the bacon, potato noodles, cream sauce, mozzarella, salt, and pepper. Allow to chill for 2 hours.

6. In a small bowl, mix the panko breadcrumbs, cumin, and remaining flour.

7. In a large, high-walled skillet or a wide-bottomed pot, heat 2 inches of oil to 325°F.

8. Using a spoon, scoop out 1-inch balls of the chilled potato and cheese mix. Coat these in the panko and flour mix. Carefully drop these breaded balls into the hot oil and fry until the coating is a deep golden brown, about 3 minutes.

Roasted Spiral Slicer "Leavings"

Leftovers can be great, but that's usually when you're talking about soup, pizza, or other take-out foods. What do you do with all those leftover spiral-izer "mushroom" pieces? You know, the long center and cap piece that is left behind? Well, this recipe is meant for those pieces. I hate to throw any-thing away. In fact, whenever we get a big head of broccoli or cauliflower, I will carefully cut the florets off, leaving a nice big stem that I can spiralize. They don't produce many noodles, but if you stockpile them and your spi-ralizer "leavings" throughout the week, you'll have the perfect collection of leftover veggies to roast up. For the pieces left behind when spiralizing I cut the top off of the stem piece and chop the top while cutting the stem in half.

This recipe was designed to be flexible and compatible with the widest array of vegetables possible. Feel free to play around with it. No leeks? Substitute a medium yellow onion. Not a fan of bacon? Try some cubed sausage or any other fatty meat.

MAKES 4 TO 6 SERVINGS

4 pieces thick bacon, chopped

1 leek, the green portion only, sliced thin

approximately 4 cups leftover veggies, spiralized on blade 2 or chopped small

3 tablespoons olive oil

salt and pepper, to taste

1. Preheat the oven to 425°F.

2. In a large pot on medium-high heat, add the bacon until it just begins to release some of its fat. Add the leeks and stir until the leeks are coated in the bacon fat.

3. Toss in the remaining veggies and olive oil. Salt and pepper to taste. Stir well to coat and cook on medium-high heat, stirring occasion-ally until the vegetables and bacon start to "sweat" or slightly soften. While they do this, line a baking sheet or 2 with parchment paper.

4. Transfer the vegetables to the baking sheets, making sure they are not crowded and no more than layer deep.

5. Roast for approximately 20 to 30 minutes or until the bacon is crisped and the vegetables are browning on their edges.

Hazelnut Parmesan Carrots

This is an unexpected side dish that never fails to please. Cooked carrots coated in a hazelnut-Parmesan butter topped with honey. This dish feels very classic yet new at the same time. The honeyed carrots are a nod to a classic American side dish, but the hazelnuts lend a distinctly European flavor.

MAKES 4 SERVINGS

1 pound carrots, peeled

2 tablespoons butter

1 cup toasted chopped hazelnuts, divided

2 cloves garlic

1 teaspoon kosher salt

¾ cup grated Parmesan cheese

⅓ cup extra virgin olive oil

2 tablespoons honey, for drizzling

1. Slice lengthwise down each carrot, cutting into its core. Do not cut all the way through. Using blade 1 of the spiral slicer, spiralize each carrot until you have tiny discs left.

2. In a large skillet on medium heat, melt the butter and add the carrots. Cook, covered, for approximately 7 to 10 minutes or until the carrots are softened but not falling apart.

3. While the carrots cook, put ¾ cup of the hazelnuts, the garlic, the kosher salt, and the Parmesan into a food processor. Chop the ingredients until they are nearly a paste. While the processor is running, slowly pour in the olive oil. You want a thin paste consistency.

4. Remove the carrots from the pan and toss in a bowl with the hazelnut mixture. Sprinkle with the remaining hazelnuts and honey.

Sweet Potato Chips

I love sweet potatoes and I love chips. Love them. Sadly for me, chips do not love me back, so I began looking for ways to get my salty-crunchy fix without all the frying. Enter the baked sweet potato chip! Plenty of recipes abound for homemade baked chips, but the spiralizer really helps to cut down on the prep time. In this recipe, it basically works as a stand-up mandolin. I like the unique shape made by the spiral slicer and find it's especially great at picking up dips.

MAKES 6 SERVINGS

2 pounds sweet potatoes

3 tablespoons olive oil

1 tablespoon Cajun seasoning blend

1 teaspoon kosher salt

2 teaspoons maple syrup

1. Preheat the oven to 250°F. Line 2 baking trays with parchment paper.

2. Cut the sweet potatoes with a knife lengthwise halfway into the center (do not cut through!). Spiralize them on blade 1. You should be getting little thin discs of sweet potato. The thinner the better!

3. Place all the chips in a large bowl. Add the remaining ingredients and toss to coat.

4. Spread the potatoes out in thin, even layers on the baking trays. It is important not to overcrowd them.

5. Bake as close to the center of the oven as possible for approximately 30 minutes or until the chips are cooked through and crispy. Check on the chips every 10 minutes and stir or rotate the pan if needed.

6. Allow to cool completely before serving.

Fried Onions and Flavored Mayonnaise

When Thanksgiving rolls around, I always used to find myself buying two boxes of the "shall not be named brand" fried onion toppings to go on the ubiquitous green bean casserole. The recipe only called for one box of the crunchy little gifts from heaven, but I would need the extra box to make up for all of my snacking. These babies are straight up-fried, but they are still better for you than the aforementioned "shall not be named brand" and one certain steakhouse chain's onion appetizer that consistently topped the charts for "the worst foods you could eat out." Stay in, make these instead, and use them sparingly on salads or indulge and dip them in some chipotle- or anchovy-infused mayonnaise (you know, for you health nuts out there!).

MAKES 2 CUPS ONIONS AND 1 CUP MAYONNAISE

For the fried onions:

vegetable oil, for frying

½ cup flour

½ cup panko breadcrumbs

1 teaspoon salt

½ teaspoon garlic powder

1 teaspoon dried mustard powder (optional)

1 large white or yellow onion, spiralized on blade 3

For the flavored mayonnaise:

1 cup mayonnaise

1 canned chipotle chile in adobo or 3 anchovy filets

1. In a medium pot, heat 3 inches of vegetable oil on medium-high until it reaches 350°F. Any hotter and you will burn the oil, any lower and the onions will not fry properly and instead will become soggy.

2. While you wait on the oil to become hot enough, mix all of the ingredients except for the onions in a large bowl. Add the onion strips and toss to coat. Use a strainer to gently shake off the excess flour mixture.

3. Fry the onions until golden brown, about 4 minutes per batch, and remove from the oil using a slotted spoon or metal strainer. Allow to rest in a paper towel–lined bowl.

4. To make the chipotle or anchovy mayo, blend all the ingredients in a food processor.

5. Serve slightly chilled.

Pickled Beets

Pickled beets are great on their own but ever since I discovered how easy they are to make, they have become a staple in my kitchen. This recipe is absolutely capable of being canned, and I do so at home often. Pickled beets are one of the quickest ways to brighten up a salad or sandwich, or to stuff into a morning omelet, and they go with warmed goat cheese like peanut butter goes with jelly. Before you pickle, however, you must roast! And if you so choose, you can stop right there, top them with some salt and pepper, and call it a day.

MAKES APPROXIMATELY 4 CUPS OF PICKLED BEETS

3 large red beets, peeled and spiralized on blade 3

4 tablespoons extra virgin olive oil

½ medium red onion, sliced thinly

½ cup white wine vinegar

2 tablespoons sugar

1 tablespoon black peppercorns, cracked

1 teaspoon salt

1. Preheat the oven to 425°F and line 2 baking trays with tin foil.

2. Spread the beet noodles over the 2 trays and drizzle with 2 table-spoons of olive oil per tray. Toss the noodles to ensure they are all coated in olive oil.

3. Place the trays in the oven and roast for 5 to 7 minutes, or until the beets are softened.

4. Allow the beets to cool and place them either in a large quart jar or in a bowl where they can sit and pickle for at least a day.

5. Add the remaining ingredients plus ½ cup hot water, shake the jar or stir the bowl to incorporate all of the flavors, and allow this pink beauty to sit refrigerated for at least 1 day before using.

Parsnip Kinpira

Kinpira *is a Japanese dish. Technically, it is a style of cooking that refers to any dish (usually root vegetables) that are sautéed and simmered. The resulting flavors are crunchy, sweet, a little spicy, and salty. While many recipes differ, they all call for soy sauce and mirin, a sweet rice-based cooking wine. My favorite version is made with parsnips, but burdock root is the most traditional. Carrots, rutabagas, and turnips are wonderful in this, as are leftover broccoli stems!*

MAKES 6 SERVINGS

1 tablespoon sesame oil

2 large parsnips, peeled and spiralized on blade 2

1 to 2 pinches red pepper flakes

2 tablespoons sake

1 tablespoon mirin

2 tablespoons soy sauce

1 tablespoon honey

1. In a medium skillet, heat the sesame oil on medium-high.

2. Add the parsnip noodles and cook for about 5 minutes, stirring to coat with the sesame oil.

3. Add the remaining ingredients to the pan and bring to a boil. Lower the heat and simmer the parsnips for 8 to 10 minutes or until there is no longer any liquid in the pan.

4. Enjoy hot or cold!

Zucchini Fritters

Zucchini fritters are a great start or side to any Mediterranean meal. Filling yet light, they go especially well with yogurt and hummus dips. I like to dip them in my soups as well.

MAKES 4 TO 6 SERVINGS

2 medium zucchinis, spiralized on blade 3, salted, drained, and chopped lightly

½ large yellow onion, spiralized on blade 2

1 medium clove garlic, minced

¼ cup chopped dill

⅓ cup all-purpose flour

1 teaspoon baking powder

1 teaspoon kosher salt

½ teaspoon freshly ground black pepper

1 egg plus 1 egg white, beaten

1. Preheat the oven to 425°F and line 2 baking sheets with parchment paper.

2. In a large bowl, mix the zucchini and onion noodles, garlic, dill, flour, baking powder, salt, and pepper. Mix in the egg and egg white, and stir until the mixture is wet and sticky.

3. Using a large spoon, shape 8 flat pancakes per tray.

4. Bake for 7 to 10 minutes or until the tops are golden brown and the fritter holds together when lifted off the tray. Gently flip and bake another 7 to 10 minutes or until the top is once again golden brown and the fritter is crisped.

5. Serve hot or at room temperature.

Savory Zucchini Bread

Classic zucchini bread is great, and by that I mean it's stupidly, wonderfully, ridiculously delightful. That being said, every time I took a bite of the sweet treat, I couldn't help but picture a rich, savory, garlic-laden version, so I came up with this recipe.

MAKES 1 LOAF

1½ cups whole wheat flour

1 cup all-purpose flour

1 teaspoon salt

2 teaspoons garlic powder

2 teaspoons baking soda

1 cup applesauce or vegetable oil, or blend of the two

4 eggs, beaten

½ yellow onion, spiralized on blade 3

1 cup shredded cheese

1 very large or 2 medium zucchini, spiralized on blade 3

½ cup sunflower seeds

1. Preheat the oven to 350°F. Spray a standard loaf pan with nonstick cooking spray.

2. In a large bowl, whisk the flours, salt, garlic powder, and baking soda.

3. In a small bowl, combine the applesauce/oil and eggs.

4. Add the egg mixture to the dry ingredients and stir until almost combined.

5. Using a spatula, fold in the onion, shredded cheese, and zucchini. Pour the batter into the prepared loaf pan. Sprinkle with the sunflower seeds, and press them slightly to ensure that they stick to the dough. Bake for approximately 1 hour, until the top is golden brown and a knife poked into the center comes out clean. Allow to cool for 5 minutes before removing from the pan. Keep stored wrapped in tin foil to maintain freshness.

CHAPTER FIVE
Casseroles

These dishes are, unsurprisingly, baked in a casserole dish. It's one of the prerequisites. If you don't have one, I thoroughly recommend you go out and buy either a 7 x 11-inch, 8 x 8-inch, or a 9 x 13-inch dish, as these are the most commonly used sizes. I also recommend glassware over metal. It allows you to watch what's happening inside. Casseroles are classic comfort food. And if you're one of those people who frowns on casseroles, don't forget—lasagna is a casserole.

Potato Gratin

Potatoes are a classic comfort food. Gratin, however, can often contain an uncomfortable amount of fat. This recipe cuts down on a lot of that fat by using milk over butter and cream, and layering the cheese throughout, so each bite has the flavor but isn't weighed down. For the potatoes, Russet is a great choice in this recipe.

MAKES 6 TO 8 SERVINGS

2 large potatoes

¾ cup milk

2 medium cloves garlic, minced

¼ teaspoon red pepper flakes

4 packed cups chopped fresh spinach leaves

pinch of ground nutmeg

salt and pepper, to taste

2 cups shredded cheddar cheese

1. Cut the potatoes lengthwise halfway to the center. Slice on blade 1 of the spiral slicer. This should leave you with little potato discs.

2. Preheat the oven to 375°F and spray a 7 x 11-inch casserole dish with nonstick cooking spray.

3. In a large skillet, heat the milk, garlic, red pepper flakes, spinach, nutmeg, salt, pepper, and potato discs. Cover and allow to simmer for about 8 to 10 minutes, or until the potato discs start to become a little tender. Remove from the heat.

4. Transfer some of this mixture to the baking dish. Spread the potatoes one layer deep. Sprinkle with some of the cheese. Repeat with the remaining potatoes and cheese, so that the top layer is coated in cheese.

5. Bake for about 40 to 45 minutes until the cheese is a nice golden brown and bubbly. Let cool for at least 10 minutes before serving.

Mexican Casserole

This recipe is a lighter version of a "Mexican Lasagna" casserole my mother would make, which used tortilla chips in place of noodles. In this recipe, I use blade 1–sliced butternut squash as the noodle/chip foundation. This dish requires very little effort and very few dishes, and it makes lots of leftovers. It's a forgiving dish that dare I say might just become an instant classic in your house. If you don't want to use chorizo, you can replace it with chunks of chicken breasts tossed in adobo chili sauce or even canned black beans. It's a rare dish that tastes this incredibly rich and flavorful without making you feel weighed down.

MAKES 8 SERVINGS

1 (3-pound) butternut squash, with as straight a neck as you can find

4 chorizo sausages or 2 (15-ounce) cans black beans with 1 tablespoon vegetable oil

1 small yellow onion, chopped

1 medium red bell pepper, chopped

salt and pepper, to taste

6 cups chopped kale

3 tablespoons salsa verde

¼ teaspoon cayenne pepper (optional)

1 cup ricotta cheese

1 egg

1½ cups shredded Monterey Jack or Mexican cheese blend, divided

sour cream and salsa, to serve

1. Peel the neck of the butternut squash and cut off a 5-inch section. Reserve the remaining squash for later. Carefully make a cut halfway into the 5-inch log, going into the center but not cutting the squash in half. Preheat the oven to 425°F.

2. Using blade 1, slice the squash by cutting into the center. You should make medallions of squash instead of one long noodle. Set these aside.

3. In a large, nonstick pan on medium-high heat, break up the chorizos. If using black beans, add 1 tablespoon of vegetable oil to the pan.

Once the oil starts to come out of the chorizo or the vegetable oil has heated up, add the onion, bell pepper, salt, pepper, kale, and the beans, if using. Cook, stirring occasionally, for 5 to 7 minutes or until all of the vegetables are softened. Set aside.

4. While the veggies are doing their magic (aka cooking), stir together the salsa, cayenne, ricotta (if using), and egg. Reserve ½ cup of the Monterey Jack or Mexican cheese blend and set it aside. Mix the remaining cheese into the ricotta blend.

5. Grease your 9 x 13-inch or similar-sized casserole dish then line it with a double layer of the squash rounds. Butternut squash can get quite soft when cooked, so a double layer helps this casserole maintain its shape. Spread a layer of the ricotta mixture on the squash and top with a layer of the chorizo/beans with vegetables. Press this all down gently so there aren't any large empty spaces. Top with butternut squash slices and repeat until you are out of the chorizo/beans with veggies and ricotta mixtures. Top with one last layer of squash and sprinkle the reserved ½ cup of shredded cheese on top. Cover with foil and bake for 35 to 40 minutes.

6. Let cool for 10 to 15 minutes before slicing. Top with sour cream or salsa to serve. This dish is excellent the second (and third) days.

Lasagna

Lasagna is classic comfort food and you'll be even more comforted making this gluten-free and veggie-filled dish! Feel free to use crumbled Italian sausage or ground beef in place of the turkey.

MAKES 8 SERVINGS

1 tablespoon extra virgin olive oil

½ medium yellow onion, diced

2 large cloves garlic, minced

½ teaspoon red pepper flakes

1 (14-ounce) can diced tomatoes

1 (6-ounce) can tomato paste

1 pound ground turkey

1 tablespoon dried oregano

salt and pepper, to taste

2 eggs, beaten

¼ cup grated Parmesan cheese

1½ cups ricotta cheese

4 medium zucchinis, spiralized on blade 1

½ cup shredded mozzarella

1. Preheat the oven to 400°F.

2. Heat the olive oil in a large skillet on medium-high. Toss the onion into the pan and cook, stirring occasionally until the onions soften and become translucent, about 5 minutes. Add the garlic and cook, stirring constantly for 30 seconds.

3. To make the meat sauce, add the red pepper flakes, diced tomatoes, tomato paste, ground turkey, dried oregano, salt, and pepper to the onion and garlic. Stir to combine everything and cook at a simmer for about 10 minutes or until the sauce is "dry" and sticks to the bottom of the pan.

4. While this is cooking, assemble the cheese mixture. In a small bowl, stir together the eggs, Parmesan, and ricotta.

5. Spray a 9 x 13-inch casserole dish with nonstick cooking spray. To assemble, lay down a layer of the zucchini noodles, top with some of the meat sauce, then top with some of the ricotta and egg mixture.

Repeat these 3 layers until you have used all the cheese and meat sauce. Top with zucchini noodles and cover those noodles with the mozzarella.

6. Bake uncovered for 45 minutes or until the cheese has begun to turn golden brown and the sauce is bubbling.

7. Once the lasagna has finished cooking, let it sit for 10 minutes, and press it down gently with a large flat spatula to release excess moisture from the zucchini. Slowly and carefully tip this out and drain the liquid, taking care not to burn yourself or dump the lasagna out.

8. Immediately cut the lasagna into portions, and if saving any for the following day, transfer the sliced portions to a plate, allowing space in between them as the zucchini may still release water.

Pastitsio

The Greeks really are onto something with their signature red sauce, if you ask me. What makes a Greek tomato sauce unique is its addition of cinnamon and bay leaves. These two ingredients add a type of heat and earthiness that is unmatched in traditional sauces from other lands. I absolutely adore it and have faith you will too. Pastitsio is the less familiar cousin to moussaka, often referred to as "Greek lasagna."

MAKES 8 SERVINGS

For tomato meat sauce:

2 tablespoons olive oil

1 medium yellow onion, chopped

2 pounds lean ground beef

½ cup dry red wine

3 large cloves garlic, minced

1 cinnamon stick

2 bay leaves

1 teaspoon dried oregano

1 (28-ounce) can crushed tomatoes, in juice

salt and freshly ground black pepper, to taste

For the noodles:

2 large zucchinis

salt

For the béchamel:

1½ cups whole milk

4 tablespoons (½ stick) unsalted butter

2 teaspoons cornstarch

¼ teaspoon ground nutmeg

salt and freshly ground black pepper, to taste

½ cup Greek yogurt

3 large eggs, beaten

1 cup freshly grated Parmesan or Kasseri cheese, divided

1. To start, make the sauce. In a large pot, heat the olive oil on medium-high. Add the chopped onion and sweat for about 5 minutes. You want them to become translucent and not take on color. Add the ground beef, breaking it up using a wooden spoon or spatula. Lower the heat to medium and cook, stirring occasionally for approximately

8 to 10 minutes or until all of the beef has browned and broken into small pieces. Turn the heat up to medium-high and add the red wine, garlic, cinnamon stick, bay leaves, and oregano. Cook, stirring constantly, for 3 minutes. Add the tomatoes, salt, and pepper. Bring to a boil, lower the heat to medium or medium-low, and simmer for about 45 minutes. Make sure to stir the sauce from time to time so that it does not stick to the bottom of the pan and burn.

2. Preheat the oven to 350°F.

3. To make the noodles, slice the zucchinis lengthwise halfway to the center, taking care not to cut all the way through. Spiralize the noodles on blade 1, salt, rest, and squeeze (page 7) to drain them of excess water.

4. To make the béchamel, heat the milk in a small pan until it just begins to simmer but does not boil.

5. In another pan, melt the butter and stir in the cornstarch on medium heat. Slowly pour in the milk, stirring constantly until the mixture begins to thicken slightly. Remove the pan from the heat. Add the nutmeg, salt, pepper, yogurt, eggs, and ½ cup of the cheese. Whisk vigorously to combine. Set aside.

6. To assemble: grease a 9 x 13-inch casserole dish that is 2 inches deep. Stir the drained zucchini noodles and remaining ½ cup of cheese into the tomato sauce and pour this mixture into the dish, making sure to press it down firmly and evenly. Top with the béchamel and bake for approximately 45 minutes or until the top is set and golden brown. Allow the pastitsio to cool for at least 5 minutes before serving.

Root Vegetable Rice and Beans

This recipe is inspired by what I used to buy in the diet frozen foods section. The brand shall remain nameless, but it came in a red box with the words "rice and beans" on it. This is a glorious, flavor-packed, preservative- and chemical-free version. It will be "wet" when you remove it from the oven, so do not worry. And if the fact that the inspiration was a diet food puts you off, do yourself a favor and give this quick-to-assemble recipe a chance before you pass judgment. You can't fail with rice and beans.

MAKES 10 TO 12 SERVINGS

1 small sweet potato, spiralized on blade 3, then riced

2 large parsnips, spiralized on blade 3, then riced

1 medium red bell pepper, diced

1 cup corn kernels (frozen is fine)

1 (10-ounce) can diced tomatoes with chilies

½ cup Spanish olives, sliced

1 (15-ounce) can black beans, drained and rinsed

2 cups Mexican shredded cheese blend, divided

1 cup green salsa (spice level of your choosing)

1 cup light cream cheese

½ cup medium yellow onion, diced

¼ cup sliced pickled jalapeños (optional)

1. Preheat the oven to 400°F.

2. In a large bowl, mix the vegetable rice, bell pepper, corn, diced tomatoes, olives, black beans, and one cup of the shredded Mexican cheese.

3. In a small bowl, mix the salsa and cream cheese. Mix this into the large bowl of vegetables. Pour the entire mixture into a 9 x 13-inch glass casserole dish. Top with the diced yellow onion and remaining cup of shredded cheese. Add the pickled jalapeños last, if using.

4. Bake the rice and beans, uncovered, on the lowest oven rack for 45 minutes or until the dish is bubbling and the cheese is a golden brown.

5. Allow to cool for at least 15 minutes before serving.

Tuna Noodle Casserole

What's more American than tuna noodle casserole? I love water-packed canned fish like tuna, farmed salmon, and brislings for their ability to deliver a low (or at least healthy) fat, protein, and a good punch of flavor.

MAKES 8 SERVINGS

1 (10.75-ounce) can condensed cream of mushroom soup (reduced fat if you prefer)

½ cup mayonnaise

½ tablespoon Dijon mustard

¼ teaspoon garlic power

¼ teaspoon onion powder

½ cup chopped celery

½ cup diced red onion

⅔ cup drained canned tuna

salt and pepper, to taste

2 medium zucchini, spiralized on blade 1

1 cup frozen peas, thawed

1 tablespoon butter, melted

2 tablespoons panko breadcrumbs

1. Preheat the oven to 400°F.

2. In a large bowl, mix the cream of mushroom soup, mayonnaise, Dijon mustard, garlic powder, and onion powder. Add the celery, red onion, tuna, salt, pepper, zucchini noodles, and thawed peas.

3. Grease a 9 x 13-inch casserole dish then add the mixture.

4. In a small bowl (or the same large bowl from before if you don't want to do extra dishes), mix the melted butter and panko breadcrumbs. Sprinkle onto the noodle mixture.

5. Bake for 5 minutes or until the crumbles are golden. Allow the casserole to cool, and serve.

CHAPTER SIX
Mains

Mains, aka entrées. These dishes are the meat and potatoes of this book. In fact, some of them feature meat and/or potatoes. These are the meals that are filling enough on their own to be called dinner, or a sturdy lunch. We're talking "rice" stuffed peppers, meatballs with pasta, and beef stroganoff all the way to the more exotic banh mi sandwiches, paella, and amazing versions of take-out favorites like pad thai and chicken lo mein. They're all here and more. With this section you can have dinner on the table in as few as 20 minutes, and there is at least one dish in here to satisfy every craving.

Garlicky Zucchini with Anchovy and Parmesan

While this dish has three main elements, it only takes one skillet and a food processor to make. The end result looks and tastes fancy enough to come out of any higher-end restaurant kitchen and it's a great way to dress up a large plate of deceptively healthy greens. If you have extra zucchini ends laying around from other spiralizing recipes, this is a great dish to add them to. Just sauté them with the rest of the vegetables toward the end and enjoy!

MAKES 4 SERVINGS

For the Parmesan crisps:

½ cup grated (not shredded) Parmesan cheese, divided

For the pesto:

3 tablespoons extra virgin olive oil, divided

4 cups chopped kale

3 anchovy fillets

2 cloves garlic

1 teaspoon salt

zest and juice of ½ lemon

For the pasta:

1 tablespoon extra virgin olive oil

1 large zucchini, spiralized on blade 3

2 cups thawed or pre-cooked broccoli florets

1 cup cannellini beans

¼ cup pitted olives

freshly ground black pepper, to taste

1. In a large skillet on medium-high heat, sprinkle ¼ cup of the grated Parmesan into a circle shape. The cheese should all melt into a solid circle. Cook for approximately 5 minutes or until the bottom has turned nice and golden brown; you don't want any white left on the bottom. Using a large, flat spatula, carefully flip the cheese disc and cook another 3 to 5 minutes or until both sides are completely

browned. Set aside on a paper towel–lined plate and repeat with the remaining Parmesan. This will make 2 large, crunchy cheese crackers.

2. In that same skillet, pour 1 tablespoon of olive oil and sauté the kale on medium-high heat until it has just wilted, about 3 to 4 minutes. Remove the kale from the heat and toss it into a food processor with the remaining pesto ingredients. Blitz in the food processor until it forms a smooth paste. Slowly add the remaining 2 tablespoons of olive oil while you process. Taste to see if you prefer more a lemon or anchovy flavor.

3. For the pasta, heat 1 tablespoon of olive oil on medium heat in the same skillet. Add the zucchini noodles, stir to coat with some of the oil, cover, and cook for 5 minutes. Remove the cover and turn the heat up to medium-high. Add the remaining ingredients and cook for another 5 minutes or until the noodles are cooked through and there is no water in the pan.

4. Add the pesto, stirring everything to coat, and serve in two hefty portions topped with freshly ground black pepper and one Parmesan crisp each.

Banh Mi Sandwiches

Banh mi sandwiches seem well poised to bypass pho as Vietnam's "new" favorite dish. In fact, this sandwich is far from new. Banh mi merely refers to types of bread, but in the US, we use the term to refer to a flavorful veggie-packed sandwich served on a fluffy French-style loaf.

MAKES 4 SERVINGS

½ pound daikon, peeled and spiralized on blade 3

1 large carrot, peeled and spiralized on blade 3

½ cup rice wine vinegar

3 teaspoons brown sugar

1 teaspoon salt

1 (24-inch) soft baguette or French bread loaf

2 tablespoons vegetable oil

½ pound extra-firm tofu, cut into ½-inch cubes

1 tablespoon fish sauce

½ teaspoon soy sauce

4 tablespoons mayonnaise

1 jalapeño, thinly sliced

½ medium sweet onion, spiralized on blade 3

¾ cup packed cilantro sprigs

1 cucumber, spiralized on blade 3

1. Preheat the oven to 350°F.

2. Toss the daikon and carrot noodles in a large bowl with the rice wine vinegar, brown sugar, and salt. Let this marinate for at least 15 minutes.

3. Cut the baguette open so it is split in half but still in one piece then cut into four pieces. Open the four pieces of bread and place them face down on the center oven rack. Toast in this manner for 5 minutes.

4. In a large skillet, heat the vegetable oil. Fry the tofu until crispy on the outside. Sprinkle with the fish and soy sauces. Stir to coat.

5. Drain the carrot and daikon noodles.

6. Brush the insides of the bread with the sauces from the tofu. Stuff the bread with the tofu, pressing down to slightly crush the tofu. Top the sandwiches with the mayonnaise, jalapeño slices, sweet onions, cilantro, cucumber, and marinated slaw. You may need to secure the sandwiches shut with toothpicks.

Rice Stuffed Peppers

In one of the kitchens where I used to work, there was a Serbian chef who introduced me to the concept of baked stuffed peppers. They're a wonderful way to package a nice, compact, yet hearty meal, and the baking brings out the sweetness of the red peppers. They also save well for lunch leftovers the following day.

MAKES 4 TO 6 SERVINGS

3 tablespoons olive oil, divided

2 medium celeriac, peeled, spiralized on blade 3, then riced

½ medium red onion, chopped

1 (14.75-ounce) can diced tomatoes, drained

1 tablespoon chopped fresh oregano

½ cup crumbled feta

¼ cup chopped fresh parsley

2 teaspoons salt

4 to 6 medium to large red bell peppers, tops cut off and hollowed out

1. Preheat the oven to 350°F.

2. In a large skillet, heat 1 tablespoon of the olive oil on medium-high heat. Add the celeriac rice and cook, covered, for 8 to 10 minutes, making sure to stir from time to time. The rice should start to soften. Remove the rice from the heat.

3. Add the chopped red onion, diced tomatoes, oregano, feta crumbles, parsley, and salt to the rice. Stir to mix all of the ingredients completely.

4. Stuff this mixture into the peppers. Place the peppers into a casserole dish, tops up, and brush the outsides of the peppers with the remaining olive oil.

5. Bake for 30 minutes or until the top of the rice begins to brown and the peppers are soft. Serve hot.

Pesto Pasta

Nothing (save for a fresh-picked tomato) captures the purely unadulterated flavor of summer like freshly made basil pesto. In this recipe, feel free to make your zucchini noodles any shape you prefer. I like the wider, fettuccine-style noodle, as it's great for holding onto all of the garlicky green goodness. The quality of your ingredients matters more than usual in this recipe, as there are so few ingredients being used. This dish is also lovely topped with a baked chicken breast.

MAKES 4 SERVINGS

4 tablespoons olive oil, divided

2 medium zucchinis, spiralized however you prefer

1 very large bunch fresh basil, leaves picked from the stems

1 large clove garlic

4 tablespoons freshly grated Parmesan cheese, divided

1 teaspoon lemon juice

½ teaspoon kosher salt

1. In a large skillet, heat 2 tablespoons of the olive oil on medium-high. Add the noodles and stir to coat the bottom. Cover and cook for 5 minutes or until the noodles begin to soften.

2. While the noodles are cooking, mix the remaining ingredients in a food processor, saving 2 tablespoons of the Parmesan to sprinkle on your finished dish. Blend until you have a smooth paste.

3. After the 5 minutes of cooking are up, remove the cover and continue to cook until the noodles are completely wilted and there is no moisture left in the pan.

4. Remove the noodles from the heat and toss in the pesto. Top with the remaining Parmesan and serve warm!

Spaghetti Bolognese

Bolognese is what I think of when people say "spaghetti" or "red sauce pasta." It's a classic Italian dish full of flavor, lycopene-rich tomatoes, and the umami powerhouse of tomato paste and bacon. While this dish is already pretty lean, feel free to use ground chicken or turkey if you are trying to avoid red meat in your diet.

MAKES 6 SERVINGS

4 tablespoons olive oil, divided

1½ pounds zucchini, spiralized on blade 3

1 medium yellow onion, diced fine

1 medium carrot, diced fine

1 stalk celery, diced fine

6 cloves garlic, minced

6 sliced smoked bacon, chopped

1 pound lean ground beef

¼ cup white wine

1 cup chicken stock

1 (28-ounce) can crushed tomatoes

2 tablespoons tomato paste

1 bay leaf

salt and freshly ground pepper, to taste

¼ cup grated Parmesan cheese, to top

1. Place 2 tablespoons of the olive oil in a large skillet on medium-high heat. Add the salted and squeezed zucchini noodles, toss to coat with the olive oil, and cover. Cook for 5 to 7 minutes or until the zucchini has wilted and cooked through. Set aside and dry the pan.

2. Add the remaining 2 tablespoons of olive oil and bring the pan back to medium heat. Add the onion, carrot, and celery and sweat the vegetables for 5 minutes, stirring occasionally. You want the carrots and celery softened and the onions to be translucent, without browning.

3. Stirring constantly, add the minced garlic and cook for another 30 seconds.

4. Add the chopped bacon and ground beef. Cook for approximately 10 minutes, making sure to stir frequently so that the beef is no longer red.

5. Add the white wine, chicken stock, crushed tomatoes, tomato paste, bay leaf, salt, and pepper. Bring this mixture to a boil. Lower the heat to medium-low and allow your sauce to cook, uncovered, at a low simmer for about ½ hour or until the bolognese has thickened. Make sure to stir the sauce every now and then to prevent it from sticking to the pan.

6. In the last 5 minutes of cooking, turn up the heat to medium-high and add the zucchini noodles to warm them and allow the sauce to stick to them.

7. Serve topped with freshly grated Parmesan cheese.

Classic Meatballs

For nearly two years I worked as the pastry chef of a meatball-based restaurant group. I went from never eating meatballs to eating them nearly daily. I love meatballs now, but I don't love how much fat is added to them to keep them moist and flavorful. This is my version of a classic.

MAKES 4 SERVINGS

1 pound 90 percent lean ground beef

1 pound ground pork

1 cup Greek yogurt

2 large eggs

½ cup breadcrumbs

¼ cup chopped fresh parsley

1 tablespoon chopped fresh oregano

2 cloves garlic, minced

2 teaspoons salt

¼ teaspoon crushed red pepper flakes (optional)

½ teaspoon ground fennel

1. In a large bowl, combine the ground meats, yogurt, eggs, breadcrumbs, parsley, oregano, garlic, salt, red pepper (if using), and ground fennel. Mix only to combine. You do not want to overmix or squeeze the meatballs too densely. Refrigerate for 1 hour.

2. Preheat the oven to 425°F. Line a baking sheet with tin foil and either rub with oil or spray with nonstick cooking spray.

3. Roll the meat into 1½-inch-diameter balls and place on the baking sheet. You can either spray your hands with cooking spray or keep a shallow bowl of water handy to keep your hands wet. This will help prevent the meat from sticking.

4. Bake the balls for approximately 20 minutes, or until the outside is browned and the internal temperature is 165°F and no longer pink.

Crawfish Pasta

I prefer uncooked zucchini noodles in this recipe. The lightness of the raw vegetable helps to carry some of the cheese in this dish, which is basically a spicy bayou mac and cheese–style meal. It's not the kind of dish that you would find in a restaurant, but it's absolutely the kind of dish you'll find in Louisiana family–style gatherings. If the ¼ cup butter is too much for you, substitute 2 tablespoons of olive oil for the onions and peppers and add 3 tablespoons of water when you add the crawfish and crab.

MAKES 4 SERVINGS

¼ cup butter

½ cup chopped onion

¼ cup chopped red bell pepper

2 cloves garlic, minced

1 (16-ounce) package cooked and peeled whole crawfish tails

½ cup uncooked crab meat

1 tablespoon Cajun seasoning blend

½ cup half and half

½ cup sliced fresh mushrooms

½ cup shredded cheddar cheese

1 teaspoon Louisiana-style hot sauce

1 teaspoon smoked paprika

3 green onions, sliced thin

1 large zucchini, spiralized on blade 1

1. In a large skillet on medium heat, melt the butter. Add the onion and pepper and cook for approximately 5 minutes or until softened. Add the garlic, crawfish tails, crab meat, and Cajun seasoning. Allow this mixture to come up to a simmer and cook for an additional 5 minutes.

2. Add the half and half, fresh mushrooms, cheddar cheese, hot sauce, and smoked paprika. Cook, stirring, until the cheese melts and the mixture thickens up, about 3 to 5 minutes. Stir in the green onions and zucchini noodles. Serve hot.

Lobster and Seafood Mélange Pasta

This pasta is an indulgent dish with a unique ingredient: chayote. Chayote is technically a fruit usually found in the "exotic" or Latin produce section of your grocery store. It's wonderfully mild with a nice crunch to it. If you can't find it you can substitute zucchini for this recipe.

MAKES 4 SERVINGS

1 (2-pound) live lobster

½ cup extra virgin olive oil

1 medium yellow onion, sliced

¼ cup butter

1 tablespoon red pepper flakes

1 cup dry white wine

1 teaspoon chopped fresh oregano

5 cloves garlic, chopped

1½ pounds littleneck or Manila clams

12 raw jumbo shrimp, peeled and deveined, tails left on

8 whole squid, cleaned and sliced

1 (28-ounce) can crushed tomatoes

1 pound chayote, spiralized on blade 2

salt and pepper, to taste

juice of 1 lemon

¼ cup roughly chopped parsley, for garnish

1. Bring a large pot of salted water to a boil and cook the lobster for about 13 to 14 minutes or until the shell turns red and the meat is soft. Remove from the water and set aside until it is cool enough to handle. Remove the meat and chop it coarsely. Set the meat aside. Drain all of the water before placing the shells back in the large pot.

2. Heat the ½ cup of oil with the shells and onion and bring them up to a simmer on medium-high heat. Cook for about 10 minutes, until the shells begin to release an aroma and turn a nice golden color, and the onions become translucent.

3. Remove the shells and then add the lobster along with the butter, red pepper flakes, white wine, oregano, garlic, clams, shrimp, squid, and tomatoes, simmering until the sauce reduces partially and the clams open up, about 7 to 10 minutes.

4. Stir in the chayote noodles and simmer another 3 to 4 minutes or until the sauce sticks to the noodles and they are slightly softened.

5. Add salt and pepper to taste, sprinkle with the lemon juice, and top with parsley to serve.

Shrimp Scampi

Here's a dish that needs practically no introduction when it comes to pasta: shrimp scampi. I like my scampi the classic way, with lots of butter, lots of garlic, and a healthy amount of lemon. Once you have everything measured out and ready, this recipe comes together in less than 15 minutes.

MAKES 4 SERVINGS

1 tablespoon extra virgin olive oil

5 cloves garlic, minced

3 medium zucchinis, spiralized on blade 3

½ cup butter, cut into cubes

1 cup dry white wine, such as Sauvignon Blanc or Pinot Grigio

juice of 1 small lemon

1 pound shrimp, peeled and deveined

2 tablespoons minced flat-leaf parsley

½ cup grated Parmesan cheese

freshly ground black pepper, to taste

1. In a large skillet, heat the oil on medium-high.

2. Add the garlic and cook, stirring constantly for 30 seconds. Add the zucchini noodles and stir to coat in the garlic and olive oil. Cook, uncovered, for about 5 minutes, or until any water from the noodles has cooked off.

3. Add the butter, stirring constantly to melt. Add the wine and lemon juice and stir to combine.

4. Add the parsley and Parmesan and cook for 5 minutes, stirring occasionally, until the shrimp turn pink and begin to curl up oh-so slightly.

5. Serve topped with freshly ground black pepper.

Chicken Lo Mein

The biggest surprise that I have discovered using the spiral slicer is how perfectly it re-creates all the not-so-good for me take-out options that I used to fall back on when I was feeling too rushed to cook. This recipe may take even less time than calling your local Chinese joint and waiting on the delivery man, and it's definitely cheaper and healthier!

MAKES 6 SERVINGS

2 tablespoons sesame oil

1 medium yellow onion, chopped

2 medium carrots, peeled and sliced thin

½ head medium white cabbage, sliced thin

1 cup sugar snap peas

4 large or 5 medium zucchinis, spiralized on blade 3

3 cloves garlic, minced

¼ cup oyster sauce

⅓ cup soy sauce, plus more to taste if needed

2 cups cooked light or dark meat chicken, cut into small pieces

1. In a large skillet, heat the sesame oil on medium-high.

2. Add the onion, carrots, cabbage, and sugar snap peas. Cook, stirring occasionally, until the cabbage is wilted and the onions begin to turn translucent, about 5 to 10 minutes.

3. Add the zucchini noodles, garlic, oyster sauce, and soy sauce. Cook until the noodles begin to soften but have not taken on the color of the soy sauce, about 5 minutes.

4. Add the chicken and stir to mix everything well. Cook, stirring more frequently as the sauce begins to thicken, so that it does not burn. The lo mein is ready once the noodles hold onto the darker color of the sauce and when the water from the zucchini noodles has cooked off.

Japchae

Japchae is a wonderful Korean stir-fry dish consisting of vermicelli noodles made out of sweet potato starch. The noodles don't taste like sweet potatoes, though, which is why zucchinis are used in this recipe.

MAKES 4 SERVINGS

7 tablespoons vegetable oil, divided

4 ounces pork shoulder, cut into ¼-inch-wide strips

2 large dried shiitake mushrooms, soaked in warm water for 2 to 3 hours and cut into thin strips (reserve ½ cup of the soaking water)

3 cloves garlic, minced

3 tablespoons soy sauce

1 tablespoon honey

2 tablespoons sesame oil

1 large zucchini, spiralized on blade 3

2 to 3 green onions, cut crosswise into 2-inch pieces

1 medium yellow onion, spiralized on blade 3

1 medium carrot, spiralized on blade 3

½ red bell pepper, cut into thin strips

4 ounces spinach, roughly chopped

salt and pepper, to taste

2 tablespoons toasted sesame seeds

1. In a large skillet, heat 1 tablespoon of vegetable oil on medium-high. Add the pork shoulder and mushrooms and cook, stirring once or twice, until the meat is browned, about 5 to 8 minutes. Set aside in a large bowl.

2. Combine the garlic, soy sauce, honey, and sesame oil. Set this sauce aside.

3. Return the skillet to medium-high heat and add 2 tablespoons of vegetable oil. Add the zucchini noodles and stir. Cover and cook until the noodles are wilted, about 7 to 10 minutes. Remove from the heat and set the noodles aside in the large bowl with the beef and mushrooms.

4. Add another 2 tablespoons of vegetable oil to the skillet and fry the green onions and yellow onion on high heat for about 2 minutes. Add to the beef and noodles.

5. Add another 2 tablespoons of vegetable oil to the skillet and fry up the carrot and bell pepper on high heat for about 2 minutes. Add to the beef and noodles.

6. Add the reserved ½ cup mushroom water to the skillet on medium-high heat and add the spinach, salt, and pepper, cooking until it is just wilted. Remove from the heat, drain, and add to the vegetable and beef mixture.

7. Pour the sauce over the bowl of meat and stir-fried veggies. Sprinkle with the toasted sesame seeds and toss to combine. Serve hot.

Beef Stroganoff

Beef stroganoff has Russian heritage, but I'm not sure how authentically Russian the modern version of the recipe that everyone is so familiar with is. I am, however, certain of how very delicious it is.

MAKES 6 SERVINGS

3 tablespoons vegetable oil

2 pounds beef chuck roast, trimmed of excess fat and cut into ½ x 2-inch strips

salt and freshly ground black pepper, to taste

1 leek, sliced thin

1 cup beef broth

3 tablespoons all-purpose flour

2 teaspoons mustard

8 ounces fresh mushrooms, sliced

2 large zucchinis, spiralized on blade 1

2 tablespoons red wine

1. In a large skillet, heat the oil on medium-high. Add the beef, salt, and pepper and cook for 1 minute on each side, just to brown the strips. Move the beef over to the side of the pan.

2. Add the leek and cook for 2 minutes or until it begins to wilt. Slide the onions over to the side with the beef.

3. Pour the broth into the pan and bring to a simmer. Add the all-purpose flour and mustard, stirring constantly. Add the mushrooms and stir the beef and leeks into the liquid. Cover and simmer for 45 minutes or until the beef is tender and the mushrooms are cooked.

4. While the beef and mushrooms are cooking, in another pan sprayed with nonstick cooking spray, cook the zucchini noodles, covered, for about 7 to 10 minutes or until they are cooked through and have released their water. Drain and set aside.

5. Add the red wine to the pan with the beef. Taste again, adding salt and pepper as needed. Stir to combine everything, and simmer, covered, for another 5 minutes before serving on top of the cooked zucchini noodles.

Porcini Pancetta Parsnip Risotto

After a trip to an intensely Italian neighborhood in the Bronx, I found myself searching for a use for dried porcini mushrooms and some fresh pancetta. Luckily, I had plenty of leftover parsnips and came up with this hearty risotto.

MAKES 4 TO 6 SERVINGS

6 slices pancetta, chopped

3 tablespoons butter

1 small yellow onion, diced

1½ pounds parsnips, spiralized on blade 3, then riced

2 cups chicken broth

¼ cup dried porcini mushrooms

2 teaspoons salt

porcini mushroom powder (optional)

NOTE: The porcini mushroom powder listed in the ingredients can be made by grinding your own dried porcini mushrooms.

1. In a large skillet, cook the pancetta until crispy. Set aside. Return the pan to the heat.

2. Melt the butter in the skillet. Once melted, add the diced onion and cook until translucent, about 5 minutes.

3. Add the parsnip rice and cook, without stirring, for another 5 minutes. You want the parsnip to begin to get a nice roasted look on the bottom.

4. Pour the chicken broth over the rice and stir. Add the dried porcini mushrooms and salt. Bring the broth to a simmer. Cook, uncovered, for approximately 15 minutes, stirring occasionally, until the parsnip rice has cooked through and the liquid has cooked off.

5. Top with pancetta and porcini powder, if using, and serve.

Paella

When I lived in Barcelona, paella was everywhere. It's a dish that used to fill me with a lot of intimidation. It was assumed you needed to buy a special pan, have on hand a laundry list of ingredients, and watch over it so that it was cooked slightly too long. Now, however, I've realized that it's merely a delicious dish that plays on some of Spain's best ingredients and is very forgiving should you overcook it slightly. So don't be afraid and give it a shot—you'll be glad you did.

MAKES 6 SERVINGS

1 tablespoon extra virgin olive oil

3 cloves garlic, minced

1 teaspoon saffron threads

1 small yellow onion, chopped fine

1 small red bell pepper, diced

4 chicken thighs

1 large chorizo sausage, cubed

1 (14.5-ounce) can diced tomatoes

1 cup frozen peas

1 large yam, peeled, spiralized on blade 3, then riced

1 teaspoon smoked paprika

12 medium shrimp, defrosted if frozen, peeled, and deveined

2 tablespoons lemon juice

½ cup chopped fresh parsley

salt and pepper, to taste

1. Pour the olive oil into a large skillet on medium heat. Once the oil is nice and hot, add the minced garlic and stir constantly for about 30 seconds. Add the saffron threads, yellow onion, red bell pepper, and chicken thighs. Stir occasionally and cook until the onions begin to turn translucent and the peppers are softened, about 3 to 5 minutes.

2. Add the chorizo and cook for another 5 minutes. Pour the tomatoes, juices and all, into the skillet. Add the peas, rice, and paprika and stir everything up. Press the shrimp into the rice dish, cover, and cook without stirring for another 5 to 10 minutes, until the bottom of the

rice sticks to the bottom of the pan and the shrimp are pink and cooked through.

3. Stir the lemon juice, parsley, salt, and pepper in a small bowl and pour over the paella. Serve immediately.

Pork Katsudon

Pork katsudon *is a very popular Japanese dish that consists of a fried pork cutlet on a bowl of rice, full of lots of onions and sometimes topped with an egg (sometimes the egg is mixed in). This recipe takes a distinctly American spin on a Japanese classic, with its addition of a honey mustard apple slaw and the use of long-grain and wild rice. This dish can easily be doubled.*

MAKES 2 SERVINGS

vegetable oil, for frying

⅔ cup panko breadcrumbs

3 large eggs, divided

2 boneless pork chops, pounded thin

1 medium yellow onion, sliced thinly

2 tablespoons apple cider vinegar

2 tablespoons honey

2 tablespoons Dijon mustard

1 red apple, spiralized on blade 3

steamed green beans, to serve on the side

2 cups hot, cooked long-grain and wild rice

1. In a large lidded skillet, heat ½-inch of oil on medium-high to fry your pork chops.

2. Place the panko breadcrumbs on a plate. Beat one of the eggs and dredge each pork chop through it, then bread each chop with panko, leaving them to rest in the crumbs while you wait for the oil to heat up. Once the oil is hot enough, fry each cutlet until it is cooked through, about 4 to 5 minutes each side. Set aside the cutlets, and dispose of the cooking oil. Return the skillet to medium-high heat.

3. Add the sliced onions and cook until soft and translucent. About halfway through, when the onions begin to stick to the bottom of the pan, add half of the apple cider vinegar, making sure to scrape all of the delicious brown bits off of the bottom of the pan. These bits contain crazy amounts of flavor and are a good thing.

4. While the onions are cooking, slice the pork cutlets into manageable strips. If the onions continue to stick to the pan use the remaining

vinegar to deglaze the pan. Once the onions are softened, place the sliced pork on top of the onions. Beat one egg and pour it on top of one of the pork chops. Repeat this with the other egg and cutlet. Cover and lower heat to medium.

5. While the eggs are cooking, mix the honey and mustard in a large bowl. Add the spiralized apples and toss to combine.

6. Once the eggs are cooked, remove the skillet from the heat, but keep the lid on.

7. To serve, assemble the katsudon in a bowl as so: Place the side of steamed green beans on one side, and fill the other half of the bottom of the bowl with the cooked rice. Top with the wilted onions and pork cutlet covered in egg. Lastly, place the honey mustard apple slaw on top, and enjoy!

Mini Greek Turkey Meatballs on Zucchini Noodles

I love the miniature nature of these feta cheese–enhanced meatballs. Each one is a tiny bite of light turkey packing a powerful Greek-flavored punch. Don't let the three-step process scare you. You can easily whip up the pesto while the meatballs cook, and the noodles merely need to get warmed before stirring everything together.

MAKES 4 SERVINGS

For the meatballs:

1 (16-ounce) package lean ground turkey

½ cup yellow onion, chopped fine

1 medium clove garlic, minced

1 tablespoon dried oregano

½ cup crumbled feta cheese

2 eggs

1 cup panko breadcrumbs

1 tablespoon extra virgin olive oil

For the pesto:

½ cup pitted kalamata olives

2 cloves garlic

1 cup fresh spinach

¼ cup extra virgin olive oil

For the pasta:

1 tablespoon extra virgin olive oil

2 large zucchinis, spiralized on blade 3

1. To make the meatballs, combine all of the ingredients in a large bowl. This may be easiest to mix by hand, as you want to ensure that you are mixing each ingredient around equally. Otherwise, a strong spatula can work.

2. In a large skillet, heat the olive oil on medium-high. Roll the meat into balls about 1 inch wide. Add the meatballs to the pan, making sure not to crowd it. Cook the meatballs in two batches if need be. Cook until the meatballs are browned on all sides and the centers are cooked through, about 5 minutes. Set the meatballs aside.

3. To make the pesto, place all of the pesto ingredients into the bowl of your food processor and process until a paste is formed. You may have to stop the processor, scrape down the sides of the bowl, and mix again.

4. To cook the noodles, using the large skillet once more, heat the olive oil on medium-high. Add the noodles, stir to coat with oil, cover, and cook for approximately 7 minutes or until the noodles are softened.

5. To serve, add the pesto to the noodles and toss to combine. Top with the mini meatballs.

Veggie Patty

A good veggie patty can help rescue you on a weeknight when you don't really feel like cooking or trying a new, involved recipe. This is a straightforward recipe that benefits from the slight sweetness of the cooked parsnips. I love this recipe paired with a strong mustard and some mayonnaise on toasted brioche buns.

MAKES 4 LARGE PATTIES

3 tablespoons butter

2 medium parsnips, spiralized on blade 3

1 pound button mushrooms, sliced thin

1 medium clove garlic, minced

1 teaspoon salt

¼ teaspoon freshly ground black pepper

4 eggs

½ cup panko breadcrumbs

1. In a large skillet, melt the butter on medium-high. Once the butter is melted, add the parsnip noodles, cover, and cook for 5 minutes.

2. Remove the cover and add the mushrooms. Stir occasionally and cook for another 5 minutes, or until the mushrooms release some of their liquid and the noodles are softened.

3. Add the garlic, salt, and pepper. Cook for 1 more minute. Remove from heat and allow to cool just enough to handle.

4. Mix in the eggs and breadcrumbs. Form patties with your hands, compacting them firmly.

5. Return the now-empty skillet to medium-high heat and cook the patties, flipping once, until they are cooked through, about 3 to 4 minutes per side.

6. Serve with your favorite burger toppings and enjoy!

Potato Noodles with Andouille and Red Beans

This noodle dish is a play on jambalaya and features some of the most well-known and best-loved flavors from the Southern Louisiana region. Andouille is a unique smoked sausage. If you cannot find it, try substituting it with a kielbasa or other smoked sausage. Alternatively, you can add a teaspoon of liquid smoke to your dish.

MAKES 4 SERVINGS

1 tablespoon salt

2 medium white potatoes, spiralized on blade 3

1 link andouille sausage, sliced

4 green onions, sliced

3 cloves garlic

2 tablespoons vegetable oil

2 teaspoons Cajun seasoning blend

1 (15-ounce) can red beans

4 cups collard greens, chopped

salt and pepper, to taste

1. Bring a large pot of water to a boil. Add the salt and then the potato noodles. Blanche (a quick cook in water) the noodles for 3 minutes. Drain the noodles and set them aside.

2. In a large skillet on medium heat, cook the andouille sausage until it begins to release some of its oil, about 3 to 4 minutes. Add the sliced green onions and cook another couple of minutes. Toss in the garlic and stir nonstop for 30 seconds. Add the vegetable oil, Cajun seasoning, and potato noodles and cook, stirring occasionally, for 5 to 7 minutes or until the potato noodles begin to take on some color.

3. Add the red beans, collard greens, salt, and pepper and cover. Cook for 5 more minutes or until the greens are wilted. Stir to mix everything together and serve hot.

Pad See Ew

While pad see ew isn't as popular as pad thai, it is just as well liked. The noodles used in this dish are flatter and broader than in pad thai. The sauce also has a deeper, richer flavor. As much as I enjoy pad thai, I find myself making pad see ew, as it requires fewer ingredients. The entire dish is ready in 20 minutes or less.

In this recipe you will find two unusual ingredients. The first is oyster sauce and there really is no substitution for this. You can find it at any Asian grocery store and at many well-stocked grocery stores. If you are allergic to shellfish, "vegetarian oyster sauce" is a perfect substitution, as it is made from mushrooms. I recommend breaking down and getting the oyster sauce. There really is no better way to up your beef and broccoli or Asian stir-fry game. The second ingredient is kecap manis, or "dark sweet soy sauce." If you do not wish to buy a bottle of this, it is pretty easy to make with items you most likely already have in your pantry. The recipe for homemade kecap manis is listed at the end of this recipe.

MAKES 6 SERVINGS

1 tablespoon vegetable oil

3 cloves garlic, minced

1 boneless chicken breast, cut into small chunks

2 eggs

1 large zucchini, spiralized on blade 3

1 head's worth of bok choy greens, chopped

For the sauce:

1 tablespoon brown sugar

3 tablespoons kecap manis or hoisin sauce

3 tablespoons oyster sauce

2 teaspoons soy sauce

2 teaspoons rice wine vinegar or white vinegar

1. In a large skillet, heat the oil on medium-high. Add the minced garlic and stir constantly for 30 seconds. Add the cut-up chicken breast and stir to coat each piece with some of the garlic oil. Allow the chicken to cook, stirring occasionally for 6 minutes.

2. While the chicken is cooking, mix your sauce. In a small bowl, stir the brown sugar, kecap manis or hoisin sauce, oyster sauce, soy sauce, and vinegar. Set aside.

3. Push the chicken to the perimeter of the pan and crack both of the eggs in the middle. Using your spatula or wooden spoon, stir up the eggs to scramble them in the center. Once the eggs are almost completely cooked through, stir the chicken into them.

4. Add the zucchini, chopped bok choy, and sauce mix. Stir to coat. Turn the heat up to high. Stir occasionally and allow the noodles to become softened and translucent. The noodles and greens will release a lot of water. Allow that water to cook down and wait for the sauce to thicken to the point that it will coat the noodles. The greens and noodles should be wilted and coated in a thickened brown sauce. This will take about 10 minutes. Serve immediately.

NOTE: To make homemade kecap manis, mix together 2 tablespoons of soy sauce and 1 ½ tablespoons of honey.

Pad Thai

Pad thai is the ubiquitous Thai stir fry. In fact "pad" is just a way of saying something that has been fried in a wok. With the number of ingredients listed here, pad thai may seem like a lot of work, but once you have every-thing measured out it goes pretty quickly. More quickly, I bet, than driving to your local Thai restaurant. Fish sauce may seem like a weird ingredient, but it essential for truly authentic Thai flavors. Just don't drop the bottle—the flavor is better than the smell, trust me.

MAKES 6 SERVINGS

2 tablespoons vegetable oil

¼ cup tamarind paste

2 tablespoons fish sauce

3 tablespoons brown sugar

1 Thai chile, seeded

2 cloves garlic, minced

2 green onions, sliced

2 boneless chicken breasts, cut into cubes

2 large eggs

1 large zucchini, spiralized on blade 2

1½ cups mung bean sprouts

chopped toasted peanuts, chopped cilantro, and lime wedges, to serve

1. In a large skillet, heat the oil on medium-high. Add the tamarind paste and stir it into the hot oil to break it up. Add the fish sauce, brown sugar, Thai chile, garlic, and green onions. Stir everything together for about 1 minute.

2. Add the chicken breasts and stir together to coat the chicken in the sauce. Stir occasionally until the chicken is almost fully cooked, about 6 minutes. Move the chicken to the perimeter of the pan and crack the eggs in the center of the pan, scrambling them with your spatula/spoon. Once the eggs are almost fully cooked, stir the chicken together with them.

3. Add the remaining ingredients and stir to combine. The noodles will release a lot of water. You want to turn the heat up to high once they do this and cook, stirring occasionally for approximately 10 minutes or

until the noodles are wilted and the sauce is thick enough to coat the noodles.

4. To serve, dish out into bowls and top with chopped peanuts and cilantro. Squeeze the lime wedge on top. Serve with extra lime wedges.

Alsatian Potato Bowl

On the handful of rare occasions when my fellow pastry school classmates and I had gotten ahead of our curriculum, our mind-blowingly talented chef instructors would introduce us to regional specialties of the areas they grew up in. One of the dishes that I will always remember is the Alsatian tart flambé. Taken down to the bare essentials, it is composed of a thinly stretched-out flat bread topped with crème fraîche, sliced onions, and bacon. So pure, so simple, so delicious, but not exactly health food. After pastry school, I moved to New York City and found myself settled in the Brooklyn neighborhood of Bushwick for a time. This seemed to be the epicenter of a small health food craze—the rice/noodle bowl. Basically, take whatever ingredients you have or are in the mood for and mix with brown rice or whole wheat noodles. This dish is my Brooklyn-influenced riff on the timeless Alsatian classic. I give you: The Alsatian Potato Bowl.

MAKES 2 SERVINGS

4 small red skinned potatoes

2 tablespoons olive oil

6 slices thick-cut bacon

2 cups thinly sliced yellow onion

½ cup mascarpone cheese

½ cup crème fraîche

salt and pepper, to taste

chives, for garnish (optional)

1. Preheat the oven to 425°F.

2. Slice the potatoes halfway to the center, lengthwise, taking care not to cut them in half, then spiralize on blade 3. Since you have sliced them halfway into the center, the noodles should automatically be shorter. If they are coming out too long, break them up by hand. Toss the noodles in the olive oil and season with salt and pepper. Spread out evenly on a sheet pan, making sure not to crowd the noodles. Place in the preheated oven on the middle rack. Roast for 20 minutes or until the tops of the noodles are softened and the bottom of the noodles are getting crisped and browned.

3. In a skillet, cook the bacon and set it aside to rest on a paper towel–lined plate.

4. Cook the onions in the hot bacon fat on medium-high heat until they are softened and translucent. Turn off the heat.

5. Once the potatoes are cooked, take them out of the oven, turn on the broiler, and return the potatoes to the oven. Broil for approximately 4 minutes, being careful not to burn them.

6. Crumble the bacon and place back in the pan with the onions. Add the potatoes to the pan and stir everything to combine. Mix together the mascarpone and crème fraîche and pour over the potato mixture. Stir well to break up any clumps of potato noodles or crème fraîche.

7. Serve immediately in a bowl. Top with chives, if using. This goes great with a nice kale salad, naturally.

Bibimbap

Bibimbap *(which means "mixed rice")* is a classic Korean dish, and this recipe features the use of bulgogi, a Korean-style marinated beef, as the main protein. Feel free to use chicken, pork, tofu, or whatever protein you prefer. Despite the long ingredient list, this is a relatively simple dish of lightly burnt rice topped with whatever you have in the kitchen and a quick sauce. Feel free to experiment and have fun!

MAKES 4 SERVINGS

For the bulgogi:

1 tablespoon soy sauce

1 tablespoon sesame oil

1 scallion, thinly sliced

1 medium clove garlic, minced

2 teaspoons brown sugar

1 teaspoon grated peeled ginger

½ pound ground beef

1 tablespoon vegetable oil

For the crisp rice:

1½ tablespoons toasted sesame oil, divided

2 medium sweet potatoes, spiralized on blade 3, then riced

For the sauce:

1 tablespoon sesame oil

1 tablespoon brown sugar

1 teaspoon garlic, minced

1 teaspoon rice vinegar

1 teaspoon red pepper flakes

Bibimbap mix-ins:

1 small zucchini, spiralized on blade 3

1 large carrot, spiralized on blade 3

4 fried eggs

kimchi

1. In a bowl, combine the soy sauce, sesame oil, scallion, garlic, brown sugar, ginger, and ground beef. Stir this until all of the liquid has mixed in with the beef. Refrigerate for a minimum of 30 minutes, or preferably overnight.

2. In a large wok or skillet, heat the vegetable oil on medium. Cook the beef, stirring occasionally for 6 to 8 minutes or until the beef is cooked through. Set aside and wipe the wok clean.

3. Add the sesame oil back on medium heat to make the crisp rice. Stir the sweet potato rice into the hot sesame oil and stir to coat. Press the rice flat and cook until the rice has crisped on the bottom, about 15 minutes.

4. While waiting on the rice to crisp, mix together the sauce. Stir together all of the ingredients and set it aside.

5. Divvy up the crisped rice into bowls. Top with the bulgogi and various mix-ins. Serve with a drizzle of the sesame sauce and top with the fried egg and kimchi. Enjoy immediately.

Indian-Style Potatoes and Chickpeas

Some days it feels like I have more spices in my cupboard than fresh food in the refrigerator. On days like these, I make Indian food. This dish is an inspired combination of palak paneer *and* sag aloo, *plus a new addition with the roasted chickpeas on top. I firmly believe you should always have canned chickpeas and frozen spinach on hand for last-minute dinners that you'll want to make again and again.*

SERVES 3

For the roasted chickpeas:

1 (15-ounce) can chickpeas, rinsed and drained and set out to dry on paper towels

2 tablespoons vegetable oil

2 tablespoons Dijon mustard

2 tablespoons mayonnaise

3 teaspoons spicy curry powder

For the spinach potato noodles:

2 tablespoons vegetable oil

1 tablespoon brown mustard seeds

1 tablespoon yellow mustard seeds

½ cup diced yellow onion

1 (10-ounce) package of frozen spinach, thawed

1 large Russet potato, spiralized on blade 3

1 cup salted ricotta cheese

1. Preheat the oven to 450°F. Line a baking sheet with parchment paper.

2. Make the roasted chickpeas. Toss the chickpeas in the vegetable oil. Spread the chickpeas out on the baking tray and roast for 30 to 45 minutes or until the chickpeas are browned and crispy. Set the chickpeas aside to cool slightly.

3. While the chickpeas are roasting, blend the mustard, mayonnaise, and curry powder in a medium bowl. Once the chickpeas have cooled, stir

them into the curry mustard-mayonnaise. Reserve the chickpeas to top the spinach potato noodles.

4. Make the spinach potato dish. This can be done during the last 20 minutes of roasting time. In a large skillet, heat the vegetable oil on medium-high. Add the mustard seeds and cook until the seeds begin to "pop" out of the pan. Add the diced onion and cook, stirring frequently until the onions are soft and translucent, about 5 minutes.

5. Add the spinach and potato noodles to the pan with ½ cup of water. Bring the water to a simmer, lower the heat to medium, and cook, covered, for 10 minutes. If the pan gets too dry, you can add a splash of water whenever needed.

6. After the 10 minutes have passed your potato noodles should be softening. Once they are, remove the cover, turn the heat back up to medium-high, and cook until the moisture in the pan has cooked off and the potato noodles are completely limp and cooked through, though not necessarily browned.

7. Stir in the ricotta cheese and cook for another couple minutes, or until the ricotta is heated and sticking to the noodles.

8. Serve this meal with the spinach mixture as the base and curried roasted chickpeas on top.

Truffle Mac and Cheese

You either love truffles or you're completely over it. If you're of the latter camp, feel free to just omit this ingredient and call it "plain 'ole mac and cheese."

MAKES 4 SERVINGS

2 tablespoons vegetable oil

1 (3-pound) butternut squash, spiralized on blade 2 and chopped into 2-inch pieces

¼ cup Greek yogurt

¼ cup roasted red peppers

2 tablespoons cream cheese

½ cup grated Parmesan cheese

1 tablespoon truffle oil

1. In a large skillet, heat the oil on medium-high. Cook the squash in the oil, stirring frequently until they are softening and almost cooked throughout, but not falling apart, approximately 5 minutes.

2. While the butternut squash is cooking, combine the Greek yogurt and roasted red pepper until completely smooth in a small food processor or blender. Add this to the squash noodles.

3. Stir in the cream cheese and Parmesan cheese. Cook, stirring frequently, until the cheese thickens and begins to bubble up.

4. Remove from the heat, stir in the truffle oil, and serve immediately.

Greek Mac and Cheese

The yogurt in this recipe helps to make it slightly lighter than most flour-thickened macaroni and cheese–type dishes. The zucchini are spiralized on the first blade to give them a better ability to hold onto the cheese sauce. I've found this blade is the best for holding sauces, at least until someone clever invents an elbow macaroni spiralizer attachment.

MAKES 4 SERVINGS

2 tablespoons extra virgin olive oil

2 medium zucchinis, spiralized on blade 1 chopped into 2-inch pieces

2 cups chopped fresh spinach

½ cup plain Greek yogurt

1 cup feta cheese

2 cups mozzarella

1 teaspoon garlic powder

1 teaspoon salt

¼ cup grated Parmesan cheese, to garnish

1 tablespoon dried oregano, to garnish

1. In a large skillet, heat the oil on medium-high. Add the zucchini noodles and cook, uncovered, for 5 minutes, or until the noodles have softened and most of their water is cooked off.

2. Add the spinach to the pan and stir, cooking for 3 minutes or until it begins to wilt.

3. Stir in the Greek yogurt, feta, mozzarella, garlic powder, and salt. Continue to stir and cook until the cheese melts and coats the noodles.

4. Cook this entire dish until the cheese sauce thickens, approximately another 7 to 10 minutes.

5. Serve topped with the Parmesan cheese and oregano.

Sushi

Sushi was an unexpected but delightful spiral-slicing discovery. Sushi is one of my favorite go-to meals to make at home when I am trying to eat healthy, as I can pack each roll with tons of veggies and I always feel very full after a roll or two. The only thing I didn't love about sushi was all the rice I was eating. With spiralized and riced vegetables, though, I can double the amount of delicious and healthy vegetables that I'm getting.

MAKES 4 TO 6 ROLLS

For the rice:

3 tablespoons mirin (sweet rice wine)

1 tablespoon sugar

2 teaspoons salt

2 large parsnips, peeled, spiralized on blade 3, then riced

For the filling:

2 small zucchini, spiralized on blade 3

1 tablespoon dark sweet soy sauce (you can use a mix of 2 teaspoons soy sauce 1 teaspoon honey)

2 tablespoons olive oil

2 cloves garlic, minced

2 cups shrimp or scallops, thawed and dried if frozen

4 to 6 toasted nori sheets (amount will depend on how much you fill your rolls)

1 avocado, halved, pitted, sliced 8 times per half

To garnish:

soy sauce, pickled ginger, and wasabi

1. Make the rice. In a large skillet on medium-high heat, bring the mirin, sugar, salt, and 3 tablespoons of water to a boil. Bring down to a simmer and add the parsnip rice.

2. Stir to coat, cover, and cook for 10 to 15 minutes or until the rice is cooked through and sticking together. Set aside and allow to cool.

3. Make the sushi. In a large skillet on medium-high heat, cook the zucchini noodles with the sweet soy sauce, stirring only to prevent

the noodles from sticking. Cook until the noodles wilt entirely and are darker. Set the noodles aside and wipe the skillet clean.

4. Return the skillet to medium-high heat and add the olive oil. Once the oil is hot, add the garlic and stir constantly for about 30 seconds or until the garlic begins to release its aroma.

5. Add the seafood and cook, stirring frequently until the shrimp are pink or the scallops begin to release liquid. Remove the seafood from the heat and allow to cool.

6. To assemble, cover one nori sheet halfway with a thin layer of the rice.

7. In the middle of the rice, place a thin layer of avocado slices, some zucchini noodles, and some seafood mixture.

8. Starting with the riced side and moving away from you, roll up the sushi, making sure to hold the fillings in. Try to roll these as tightly as you can. This does take some practice, but once you have it figured out, it will be a breeze.

9. Slice with a serrated knife and serve with soy sauce, pickled ginger, and wasabi.

Butternut Squash, Browned Butter, and Sage

I'm going to make a confession here. I think the best pasta recipes are the ones that don't call for red sauce. In particular I'm thinking of butternut squash raviolis coated in browned butter and sage with a touch of Parmesan cheese. If you're thinking that this is an awful lot of butter for one recipe, well, it kind of is. But this makes a large bowl of pasta and you're putting it on top of vitamin-rich kale and butternut squash, so it all evens out right? Of course it does.

MAKES 2 TO 4 SERVINGS

1 tablespoon olive oil

½ cup yellow diced onion

4 cloves garlic, minced

½ large butternut squash, peeled and spiralized on blade 3

7 large leaves lacinato (dinosaur) kale, roughly chopped

4 tablespoons butter

¼ cup grated Parmesan cheese, plus more for topping

salt and pepper, to taste

1. In a large skillet, heat the olive oil on medium-high. Add the onions and sauté until the onions are softened and translucent, but not caramelized, about 7 minutes. Add the garlic and cook, stirring constantly until the garlic releases its aroma, about 30 seconds.

2. Add the squash noodles and stir to mix the garlic and onions into the pasta. Cover and cook, stirring occasionally, about 5 minutes. Add the kale. Stir and cover, continuing to cook for another 5 minutes. After a total of 10 minutes, the noodles should be cooked through and the kale should be wilted with a slight crunch at the rib.

3. In the meantime, in a small skillet, start to melt the butter on medium heat. Get the butter fully melted once the noodles are halfway cooked.

4. Once the noodles are cooked, turn off the heat. Raise the heat on the butter and brown the butter. Browning butter means cooking it until the color of the foam goes from white to tan. Turn off the heat once this happens or you run the risk of having blackened butter, which is burnt. The butter will continue to cook in the pan and should start to smell deliciously nutty. Once you can see small brown flecks in the butter and it has filled the room with a toasted aroma, it is ready. Immediately add it to the pasta.

5. Add the ¼ cup of Parmesan cheese, salt, and pepper. Toss to combine everything and serve topped with extra sprinkles of Parmesan cheese.

Quesadillas

Quesadillas are one of my favorite foods and always a crowd pleaser. The spiral-sliced vegetables are a great way to cut down on the amount of cheese (and therefore fat) that is typically found in this dish. This is guaranteed to please even the pickiest eater.

Epazote is an herb commonly found in Mexican cooking. Its unique flavor comes off like a cross between mint, tarragon, and citrus.

MAKES 4 QUESADILLAS

2 tablespoons olive oil, divided

1 small to medium sweet potato, spiralized on blade 3

1 teaspoon dried epazote

½ medium yellow onion, spiralized on blade 3

1 medium red bell pepper, sliced into long thin strips

2 teaspoons salt

8 medium tortillas

1 cup queso fresco

½ cup spinach, chopped

1. In a large skillet on medium, heat 1 tablespoon of the olive oil. Add the sweet potato noodles and epazote, stir to coat, cover, and cook for 5 to 7 minutes or until the noodles are soft and limp. Set them aside.

2. Returning the skillet to medium heat, add the remaining tablespoon of olive oil. Cook the onion and red pepper strips with the salt, stirring occasionally until the vegetables are soft and the onion is almost clear. Set these aside.

3. Wipe the skillet clean and spray with nonstick cooking spray. To assemble, lay down one tortilla and sprinkle with ¼ cup of the queso fresco, then top with the sweet potato noodles, onions, peppers, and some of the spinach. Top with another tortilla and gently press down. Once the bottom tortilla is nice and toasted and the cheese has melted, flip the tortillas and cook until the bottom turns golden brown. Repeat with the remaining ingredients. Serve hot.

CHAPTER SEVEN
Desserts

Surprised to see a desserts group in a book dedicated to a vegetable slicer? Don't be! The desserts in the book are the real deal—everything from the apple and oat crisps to the apple kugel to the pear bread pudding is sweet and satisfying in the way that only dessert can be. The more indulgent fruit salads have been included in this area (anything with chocolate added to it is automatically considered indulgent in my book). The use of heart-healthy fruits to add sweetness and fiber to these dishes makes them a lot less guilt inducing and a whole lot more smile inducing.

Apple and Oat Crisps

Apples love to be baked, and baked apples love to be paired with oats. If you're feeling especially indulgent, you can top this whole shebang off with some whipped cream or caramel sauce. This crumble is guaranteed to make your entire home smell amazing.

MAKES 6 TO 8 SERVINGS

3 firm apples, any color, spiralized on blade 2

1 tablespoon honey

2 teaspoons lemon juice

1 cup dark brown sugar

¾ cup oats (not instant)

¾ cup all-purpose flour

2 teaspoons ground cinnamon

¼ cup plus 2 tablespoons cold butter, cut into small cubes

1. Preheat the oven to 350°F.

2. Place the apple noodles in a large bowl, drizzle with the honey and lemon juice, and stir to coat. Place this apple mixture into a 9 x 9-inch baking dish. Press the noodles down so that they are packed and even.

3. In a food processor, mix the brown sugar, oats, flour, and cinnamon. Add the butter cubes and pulse until the mixture forms rough crumbs.

4. Spread the oat mixture evenly over the apples, pressing down on them oh-so slightly so that they attach to the apples.

5. Bake in the oven until the oat crumbles turn a nice deep golden brown and the apples have released some of their juices and begin to bubble, about 45 minutes.

Tzimmes

Tzimmes were a recent and welcoming discovery. To the uninitiated, they are more or less the Jewish version of overly sweet sweet potatoes. While tzimmes are normally a carrot dish, I like to mix mine with sweet potatoes to change it up a bit. Tzimmes (pronounced tsi-miss) are always sweetened and full of dried fruits. They are a Jewish tradition meant to symbolize a sweet and prosperous new year. The spiralizer saves the time of meticulously chopping and gets you on your way to enjoying a sweet new year or new week, or just a sweet new dish!

MAKES 8 SERVINGS

1 large sweet potato, spiralized on blade 3

1½ pounds butternut squash, spiralized on blade 2

4 large carrots, spiralized on blade 3

2 tablespoons butter

¾ cup dark brown sugar

¼ cup honey

zest of 1 orange

2 cups fresh-squeezed orange juice

2 large cinnamon sticks

⅛ teaspoon ground cloves

1 teaspoon salt

1 cup chopped prunes

1 cup raisins

1. In a large skillet with a lid, place all of the noodles and the butter. Cook on medium heat for approximately 5 minutes or until the butter coats all of the noodles and some of the noodles begin to wilt.

2. In a small bowl, mix the sugar, honey, orange zest, and juice. Add to the skillet and turn the heat up to medium-high. The liquid should start to simmer.

3. Add the cinnamon sticks, cloves, salt, prunes, and raisins and cover, allowing to cook for 10 minutes, stirring every 5 minutes.

4. After 10 minutes, remove the cover and cook for another 5 to 10 minutes or until the noodles are softened completely and the sauce has thickened enough to coat them.

5. Serve warm.

Pear Walnut and Chocolate Salad

This recipe, aside from being absolutely delicious, has the added bonus of homemade "magic shell" chocolate sauce. You will have some left over and it's great on ice cream, or anything cold. "Magic shell" is that chocolate topping you find in grocery stores that is liquid in the bottle but hardens when it comes in contact with anything cold. It is then a delightful crunchy little treat! It's similar to the German treat ischoklad, or "ice chocolate," due to the fact that it melts in your mouth like ice. This recipe makes more than you need so you will have extra. And what goes better together than pears, chocolate, and walnuts? I can't think of any reasons not to make this recipe.

MAKES 2 SERVINGS

For the salad:

1 large softened ripe pear, spiralized on blade 1

¼ cup walnuts, toasted and chopped

¼ cup chocolate sauce

sprinkle of sea salt, to taste

For the chocolate sauce:

¼ pound dark bitter chocolate, at least 70 percent cocoa, chopped up

⅔ cup coconut oil (refined is best but any will do), melted

2 tablespoons corn syrup

1. Put the pears in a large bowl and place it in the freezer to hold while you make the chocolate sauce.

2. Make the sauce. In a small microwave-safe bowl, combine the chocolate and coconut oil. Microwave on high in 10-second increments, stirring with a fork after each time until the chocolate is completely melted and combined with the coconut oil. Drizzle in the corn syrup while stirring with the fork to combine. If at any point the chocolate sauce becomes too thick, pop it back in the microwave for another 10 seconds.

3. Once the chocolate sauce is mixed and a nice, thin, pourable consistency, take the pears out of the freezer. Using your fork, gently drizzle a small amount of the chocolate sauce over the pears. Sprinkle with walnuts and a hint of sea salt. Allow the sauce to harden. If it does not within 30 seconds, place it in the freezer for 1 minute. Remove from the freezer and stir the salad, breaking up the chocolate pieces. Repeat 2 more times. Serve chilled.

Chestnut Pear Parfaits

This recipe calls for two somewhat unusual ingredients: sweetened chestnut puree and candied chestnuts. You can't make the recipe without them, but you can make your own sweetened chestnut puree by blending candied chestnuts in your food processor until utterly and completely smooth. You can find candied chestnuts in larger grocery chains and high-end kitchenware stores, especially around the holidays. Pears and chestnuts are one of my favorite flavor pairings and they almost—almost—make me look forward to winter.

MAKES 4 SERVINGS

1 cup heavy cream, chilled

7 tablespoons sweet chestnut puree, divided

2 ripe Bartlett pears, spiralized on blade 2

½ cup candied chestnuts, chopped

1. Make the chestnut cream. Beat the heavy cream with a whisk until stiff peaks form. Place 3 tablespoons of the chestnut puree in a small bowl. Spoon a small amount of the whipped cream into the bowl of chestnut puree and beat these 2 ingredients together until the puree has broken up and mixed completely with the cream. Once your cream and puree are a smooth and soft texture, *gently* fold the flavored cream into the whipped cream until just incorporated.

2. To serve, fill the bottoms of four fluted glasses or small mugs with a tablespoon of chestnut puree each. Evenly distribute the pear noodles among all the glasses and press them down to pack them in somewhat firmly. Top the noodles with the candied chestnuts and top the whole shebang off with the chestnut whipped cream.

3. Serve chilled. These can be assembled up to 1 hour in advance.

Apple Noodle Kugel

This dish is either very familiar or completely foreign to you. Noodle kugels are a Jewish dessert casserole made from either egg or potato noodles cooked in custard. As creamy and decadent tasting as they are, I was never a huge fan—that is, until I tried swapping the egg noodles out for big juicy ribbons of apples. Now the dish has a light and natural-tasting sweetness to it. Top with a sprinkle of cinnamon or cinnamon sugar, and you can't go wrong. L'chaim!

MAKES 10 SERVINGS

6 tablespoons butter, melted

1 pound cottage cheese

1 (4-ounce) package cream cheese, softened

2 cups sour cream

½ cup brown sugar

6 eggs, beaten

1 teaspoon ground cinnamon, plus more for serving

1 tablespoon vanilla extract

1 teaspoon salt

½ cup golden raisins

3 tart green apples, spiralized on blade 1

1. Preheat the oven to 375°F and spray a 9 x 13-inch casserole dish with nonstick cooking spray.

2. In a large bowl, combine all of the ingredients except for the raisins and apples. Whisk to combine. Using a large spatula, gently fold in the raisins and apple noodles, taking care not to break up all of the apple noodles.

3. Pour the mixture into the casserole dish and flatten the top, if necessary, with the spatula. Bake for approximately 45 minutes or until the top of the kugel is golden brown and the custard is no longer liquid. You do not want to see a bunch of cracks in the top of your custard; this means that you are overbaking it.

4. Allow the custard to cook for 15 minutes before cutting it. Sprinkle with a topping of cinnamon or cinnamon sugar right before serving.

Parsnip Cake

Parsnip cake is the next carrot cake. This is a wonderful way to face cold, gray winter mornings, or it can be a tasty fall harvest brunch dish. You want to use the darkest maple you find, as it packs in more maple flavor than the lighter varieties.

MAKES 10 TO 12 SERVINGS

For the cake:

2 cups all-purpose flour

1½ cups granulated sugar

½ cup dark brown sugar

2 teaspoons baking soda

1 teaspoon baking powder

1 teaspoon salt

1 teaspoon ground cinnamon

1 teaspoon ground nutmeg

4 large eggs, beaten

1 cup applesauce, vegetable oil, or a blend of the two

4 large parsnips, spiralized on blade 3, then riced

For the maple glaze:

1 cup powdered sugar

¼ cup dark maple syrup, plus more if needed

2 tablespoons softened butter

1. Preheat the oven to 350°F. Butter and flour a glass 9 x 13-inch baking pan.

2. Mix the flour, sugars, baking soda and powder, salt, and spices in a large bowl.

3. In a small bowl, mix the eggs and applesauce/oil. Add this to the large bowl of dry ingredients.

4. Fold in the riced parsnips and stir until just combined.

5. Bake on the middle oven rack until a knife poked into the center comes out clean, about 20 to 25 minutes. Allow the cake to cool completely before glazing.

6. While the cake is cooling, whisk the powdered sugar into the maple syrup in a small bowl. Beat the softened butter into the maple mix. Add more maple if you need to make the glaze a pourable consistency. If your glaze is too soft, allow it to sit for 10 minutes before stirring and if it is still too soft, add more powdered sugar, 1 tablespoon at a time until you have a thick but pourable glaze.

7. Coat the cake with a layer of the glaze and allow it to set before serving. Serve at room temperature.

Raw Fruit Tart

There was a time a while ago that I was a devout raw foodist. The biggest takeaway from that time was the amazing amount of flavor and sheer simplicity made possible in the world of raw food desserts. If you are looking to avoid gluten, dairy, eggs, and processed foods, then this is definitely the way to go for you. Don't be fooled, however—the amount of nuts definitely adds enough fat that you don't want to eat this entire pie in one sitting. But the protein from the nuts is what makes this one of my favorite breakfasts. You want to make sure the dates used in the recipe are soft and sticky; if they are not; soak them in hot water for 15 minutes and drain.

MAKES 8 SERVINGS

For the crust:

10 medium medjool dates, pitted

2 cups raw almonds

¼ teaspoon sea salt

¼ cup coconut oil, melted

For the filling:

1 cup cashews

½ cup agave nectar, plus more for optional drizzling

1 apple or pear, spiralized on blade 3

1 teaspoon vanilla extract

1 teaspoon lemon juice

pinch of ground cinnamon

1. In a food processor, grind the dates, almonds, and salt until a "dough" is formed. You want the almonds and dates to be chopped into a consistent size and for all of the ingredients to start binding together. Stop before it becomes almond butter. Move this mixture to a large bowl. Mix in the melted coconut oil by hand.

2. Press the crust mix into a 9-inch pie pan—glass works best. You want the bottom and sides to be ⅛-inch thick. Make sure to press the crust out all the way up the sides of the pan. Place the crust in the freezer for at least 20 minutes.

The **Veggie Spiral Slicer** Cookbook

3. While you wait on the crust to set, place the cashews and agave in the food processor and process until it becomes smooth and resembles custard.

4. Toss the apple or pear noodles with the vanilla, lemon juice, and cinnamon.

5. To assemble, remove the crust from the freezer and spread the cashew custard evenly over the bottom of the pie. Gently press in the apple or pear noodles on top of the custard, and if so desired, drizzle with a hint of agave. Store in the refrigerator.

Pear Bread Pudding with Bourbon Whipped Cream

This dessert sounds a lot more decadent than it actually is. Bread pudding often walks a fine line between dried out and custard. This dessert will only be as good as your pears are. By taking care to use very ripe pears, you can get away with using less fat. The juice from the fruit will keep this cake nice and moist. I substituted a traditional bourbon caramel sauce for a spiked whipped cream, which cuts both fat and sugar! If you're not calorie counting, this bread pudding is great as a breakfast the following morning, sliced and pan-fried like French toast. Just don't tell your dietitian.

MAKES 10 SERVINGS

For the bread pudding:

5 eggs

½ cup brown sugar

1 to 1½ cups milk

2 teaspoons vanilla extract

1 teaspoon ground cinnamon

¼ teaspoon salt

3 very ripe pears, skins on, spiralized on blade 2

4 cups 1-inch bread cubes (minimum 1-day-old sandwich or artisanal plain breads)

¾ cup golden raisins

For the spiked whip cream:

1 cup heavy whipping cream, chilled

1 tablespoon granulated sugar

1½ tablespoons high-quality bourbon, chilled

1. Preheat the oven to 350°F. Grease a 9 x 13-inch casserole dish.

2. In a large bowl, whisk the eggs, brown sugar, milk, vanilla extract, cinnamon, and salt, making sure there are no lumps of brown sugar. Whisk until the mixture begins to lighten.

3. Add the pears, bread cubes, and raisins. Stir a few times to make sure everything is coated in the egg mixture. You do not want to stir too much, though, as the pear noodles are fragile.

4. Gently press all of the ingredients into the prepared casserole dish.

5. Bake for 40 to 45 minutes or until the top is golden brown and the custard has gone from liquid to set. Allow the bread pudding to cool for at least 10 minutes.

6. While the bread pudding cools, make the whipped cream. Using a large bowl and a whisk, whisk the chilled heavy cream until soft peaks form. Sprinkle the sugar over the whipped cream and continue to whisk until the peaks become stiff. Gently fold in the bourbon.

7. Serve the bread pudding either warm or at room temperature. Top with whipped cream.

NOTE: Warm bread pudding will melt the whipped cream so you can serve the whipped cream on the side if serving the bread pudding warm.

Sticky Rice with Honeyed Mango

The ability to make rice-free "rice" is one of my favorite tricks of the spiralizer and one of my favorite things to do with rice is make sticky rice. Mangos are notoriously annoying to cut and peel and difficult to find perfectly ripe when you want it most. This is why I like to have frozen mangos on hand at all times.

MAKES 4 SERVINGS

For the honeyed mango:

2 cups frozen mango chunks

2 tablespoons honey

juice and zest of ½ orange

For the sticky rice:

1 yellow plantain, sliced on blade 3, then riced

1 (14-ounce) can light coconut milk

3 tablespoons sugar

½ teaspoon ground cinnamon

1. In a medium saucepan, combine all of the ingredients for the honeyed mango. Bring to a boil on medium-high heat. Reduce heat and simmer, stirring occasionally for 10 minutes. Set aside and rinse the sauce pan.

2. In the saucepan, combine all of the ingredients for the sticky rice. Bring to a boil on medium-high heat and continue to simmer for 15 minutes, stirring frequently once the milk has thickened and reduced. The rice should get so sticky that when stirred, the pudding does not immediately flood the bottom of the pan.

3. Serve layered with the honeyed mango on top of the sticky rice, warm or at room temperature.

Conclusion

The spiral slicer is a tool that is here to stay. With this book I hope that I have shown you more uses than you ever imagined. But don't stop here! Experiment with flavors that you know and love. Try and vegetize your favorite pastas, fruit-based baked goods, or salads. This wonder tool helps us remove fat and simple carbohydrates from our meals while adding texture, color, and fun! Stay hungry, stay healthy, stay happy, and never stop exploring.

—Kelsey Kinser

Conversion Charts

Volume Conversions

U.S.	U.S. equivalent	Metric
1 tablespoon (3 teaspoons)	½ fluid ounce	15 milliliters
¼ cup	2 fluid ounces	60 milliliters
⅓ cup	3 fluid ounces	90 milliliters
½ cup	4 fluid ounces	120 milliliters
⅔ cup	5 fluid ounces	150 milliliters
¾ cup	6 fluid ounces	180 milliliters
1 cup	8 fluid ounces	240 milliliters
2 cups	16 fluid ounces	480 milliliters

Weight Conversions

U.S.	Metric
½ ounce	15 grams
1 ounce	30 grams
2 ounces	60 grams
¼ pound	115 grams
⅓ pound	150 grams
½ pound	225 grams
¾ pound	350 grams
1 pound	450 grams

Temperature Conversions

Fahrenheit (°F)	Celsius (°C)
200°F	95°C
225°F	110°C
250°F	120°C
275°F	135°C
300°F	150°C
325°F	165°C
350°F	175°C
375°F	190°C
400°F	200°C
425°F	220°C
450°F	230°C

Acknowledgments

I would like to thank my patient mother for helping me to test these recipes and my wonderful boyfriend for eating all of them.

About the Author

Kelsey Kinser is a classically French–trained pastry chef and cookbook author who lives and works in New York City. After a couple years of working in fine dining restaurants in New York, she left the United States to spend a year traveling through Europe learning how to cook regional specialties. When not working she likes to make and can jam and spend too much time on the internet.